VITAL HEALTH FACTS
AND
COMPOSITION OF FOODS
for better health

CONTENTS

1-800 Hotlines to Free Health and Support Information	3
Preface	11
Understanding the Composition of Foods	13
Eating the Proper Amount of Calories-Weight Control	15
Nomogram to Estimate Calories Needed	17
Vitamin & Mineral Deficiencies - Related Health Problems	19
Supplements	21
Vitamins and Minerals - Functions and Sources	23
The Importance of Fiber	29
Fiber Content of Some Foods	31
Water - An Ultimate Substance	32
The Saturated Fat and Cholesterol Connection	33
Exercise	35
Composition of Foods/Nutritive Value of Foods Table	39

Edward A. Krimmel, BS
Patricia T. Krimmel, BSN
Directors of HELP, the Institute for Body Chemistry

Preface by Kathy A. Detweiler, M.A., R.D.
Registered Dietitian

Charles A. Krimmel
Illustrator

FRANKLIN PUBLISHERS   Box 1338, Bryn Mawr, PA 19010

This book is not intended to replace or substitute in any way the services of a physician or dietitian/nutritionist. Any application of the recommendations set forth in the following pages is at the reader's discretion and sole risk.

ISBN 0-916503-06-2   Printed in the U.S.A.

1-800 HOTLINES TO FREE HEALTH INFORMATION AND SUPPORT

All information concerning the 800 numbers should in no way be construed as an endorsement, real or implied, by the authors. Beware that some information organizations are set up as a means of getting business from you rather than giving you helpful information. In compiling the following list, we have tried very diligently to avoid all such organizations.

AIDS Hotline, National 800-342-2437, TTY/TDD, 800-243-7889, M-F, 10am-10pm ET. Information on the prevention and spread of AIDS. Referral services.

AIDS Hotline, National Indian 800-283-2437. Provides printed material and information about AIDS and AIDS prevention in the Indian community.

AIDS Clinical Trials Information Service 800-874-2572, TTY/TDD 800-243-7012. Current information on clinical trials for AIDS patients and others with HIV infection.

AIDS Information Clearinghouse, National 800-458-5231. Provides publications, and refers callers to local Information numbers on AIDS and treatment sources.

Alcoholism & Drug Dependence, National Council on 800-622-2255, 24 hours. Refers to local affiliates for counseling and provides written information on alcoholism, especially teenage drinking.

Alcohol and Drug Information, National Clearinghouse for 800-729-6686, TTY/TDD, 800-487-4889. Offers publications on prevention and education.

Al-Anon Family Group Headquarters 800-356-9996 Provides printed materials specifically aimed at helping families dealing with the problems of alcoholism.

Alzheimer's Disease Association 800-272-3900; TDD 312-335-8882. Answers questions and provides referrals to local chapters and support groups. Offers information on publications available from the association.

Amyotrophic Lateral Sclerosis Association 800-782-4747. Offers help and information to individuals with ALS and their families.

Arthritis Foundation Information Line 800-283-7800. Provides publications and information about arthritis and referrals to local organizations.

Asthma Center, National 800-222-5864. Nurses answer questions about asthma, emphysema, chronic bronchitis, allergies, juvenile rheumatoid arthritis, smoking and other respiratory and immune system disorders.

Birth Defects - March of Dimes 914-428-7100, 1275 Mamaroneck Ave., White Plains, NY 10605. Referrals to prenatal care programs, support groups, provides literature. Campaigns for healthier babies thru community services.

Blind and Handicapped, National Library for the 800-424-8567. Borrowing services of large, Braille, talking and music books.

Breast Cancer Organization, Y-ME National 800-221-2141. Provides presurgery counseling, treatment information, peer support and other services. Newsletter.

Burns Survivors, Phoenix Society for 800-888-2876. Selfhelp for burn survivors and families. Conducts school program for burned children returning to classes. Burn camps, burn congress, free care and newsletter.

Cancer Foundation, Candlelighter Childhood 800-366-2223. Offers guidance and emotional support for families of children with cancer and identifies patients and family needs to enable medical and social systems to respond adequately.

Cancer Information Service 800-422-6237, 9am-7pm Provides in depth information on all types of cancers; has second opinion panels of experts setup throughout the nation for suggesting the best care; Physician Data Base with information about every cancer specialist institution nationwide and ongoing "clinical trials". Provides supportive counseling per phone.

Cancer, National Black Leadership Initiative on 800-262-5429, Supports community cancer projects. Increase cancer prevention, education and control activities to reduce cancer mortality in the black population.

Cancer, Prostate - Us Too, Inc. 800-828-7866. Refers to peer support groups throughout United States for men with prostate cancer and their families

Cancer Research, American Institute for 800-843-8114. Provides educational resources regarding diet, nutrition, and the prevention of cancer.

Cancer Response Line, American Cancer Society 800-227-2345. Provides publications and information about cancer and coping. Refers callers to local chapters of the American Cancer Society for support services.

Celiac Disease Foundation 213-654-4085. P.O. Box 1265, Studio City, CA 91614-0265. Provides services and support to persons with celiac disease and dermatitis herpetiformis; telephone information referral services and newsletter.

Celiac Society/Dietary Support Coalition, American (ACS) 201-325-8837, 58 Musano Court, West Orange, NJ 07052. Offers counseling to people with celiac sprue. Provides information packet and quarterly newsletter.

Celiac Sprue Association/United States of America Inc. (CSA) 402-558-0600, P.O. Box 31700, Omaha, NE 68131-0770. Provides information and referral services. Quarterly newsletter.

Celiac. See Gluten Intolerance Group

Cerebral Palsy Association, United 800-872-5827. Provides packet of general information. Family counseling. Refers to local affiliates.

Children with Disabilities - National Information System and Clearinghouse 800-922-9234. Provides information on services for children to 3 years old with disabilities and does referrals to support groups, organizations, hospitals and research centers.

Child Abuse Hotline, National 800-422-4453. Provides crisis intervention and professional counseling. Refers to local agencies and supplies literature.

Child Abuse and Neglect, National Resource Center on 800-227-5242. Refers callers to specific resources in their local area and provides statistics about child abuse.

Childbirth Education Association, International (CEA) 800-624-4934. Provides referrals to local chapters, support groups, and mail order service.

Cleft Palate Association, American 800-242-5338. Information to parents and health professionals on cleft lip and cleft palate. Makes referrals to local support groups and supplies parents with list of cleft palate teams in their state.

Crippled Children, Shriners Hospital for 800-237-5055, 24 hours. Provides no-cost orthopedic and burn care for children under 18 years of age.

Cystic Fibrosis 800-344-4823. Responds to patient and family questions and offers literature. Provides referrals to local clinics.

Deaf Children, American Society for 800-942-2732. Provides support, information, referrals and encouragement to parents. Parent support network; resource materials.

Deafness - Tripod Grapevine 800-352-8888 voice/TDD, in CA. 800-287-4763 voice/TDD. Offers information on deafness, including raising and educating a deaf child. Referral to parents, professionals and resources in their own communities.

Depressive Illness, National Foundation 800-248-4344. Packet of information and referrals.

Diabetes Association, American 800-232-3472. Provides literature, information on health education and refers to local affiliates for support-group assistance.

Diabetes Foundation International Hotline, Juvenile 800-533-2873. Provides counseling and support services to juvenile diabetics and their families. Parent counseling. Refer to local chapters.

Dietetic Hotline, American 800-366-1655, 9am-4pm, ET. Questions concerning nutrition are answered by dietitians. Recorded message.

Disabilities, National Center for Youth with 800-333-6293, 8am-4:30pm CT. Information and resource center with focus on adolescents with chronic illnesses and disabilities. Helps guide youth thru transition from adolescence to adulthood.

Down's Syndrome Congress, National 800-232-6372. Answers questions about all aspects of Down's Syndrome, refers to local organizations. Newsletter.

Down's Syndrome Society Hotline, National 800-221-4602. Offers information on Downs syndrome and gives referrals to local programs for the newborn. Free information packet on request.

Drug Abuse, National Institute on 800-662-4357. Information on drug abuse and AIDS as it relates to intravenous drug users. Refers to drug rehabilitation centers.

Dyslexia Society, Orton 800-222-3123. Provides, through 44 branches, information on testing, tutoring and computers to aid those with dyslexia and related disorders.

Endometriosis Association 800-992-3636. 24 hour recording for callers to request information, leave name and address.

Epilepsy Foundation of America 800-332-1000, 24 hours. Provides information on epilepsy and makes referrals to local chapters.

Eye Care, National 800-222-3937, 24 hours. Offers medical eye care at no out of pocket expense to help those who are financially unable to visit an ophthalmologist. Must be U.S. citizen or legal resident.

Eye Research Foundation, National 800-621-2258, 24 hours. Offers printed information and referrals.

Eyes - National Center for Sight 800-331-2020 Information about eye health and safety issues and vision care through informational and fact sheets and brochures.

Gluten Intolerance Group of North America (GIG) 206-325-6980. P.O. Box 23053, Seattle, WA 98102-0353. Instructional and general information materials, as well as counseling and access to gluten-free products and ingredients; operates telephone information and referral service; newsletter.

Grief Recovery Institute 800-455-4808, 9am-5pm, PT. Provides counseling on coping with loss. Has 1200 outreach groups.

Headache Foundation, National 800-843-2256. Information and refers to local support groups.

Head Injury Foundation Family Helpline, National 800-444-6443, 9am-5pm, ET. Dedicated to improve the quality of life of people with head injury and their families.

Health Assistance Foundation, American 800-437-2423 Funds research for Alzheimer's Disease, Heart and Glaucoma. Gives financial assistance to alzheimer's patients and their caregivers through Alzheimer's Foundation Relief Program. Free publication.

Hearing Institute, Better 800-327-9355. Provides information about hearing loss, aid for the hearing impaired and is intermediator of consumer grievances.

Heart Association, The American 800-242-8721 Literature, refers to local support groups. Education and cooking programs.

Hemophilia Association, National 800-424-2634 Refers to treatment centers, chapters and support groups in callers area. Newsletter

Hospice Association, National 800-658-8898 Information about hospice care for terminally ill persons in the home and referrals to local programs .

Hospice Education Institute, Hospice Link 800-331-1620. Offers general information about hospice care and makes referrals to local programs.

Hospice International, Children's 800-242-4453, 24 hours. Within a community, provides support system and information for health care professionals, families and the network of organizations that offer hospice care to terminally ill children.

Huntington's Disease Society of America 800-345-4372. Information and referral services available for genetic counseling and other needs. Support groups.

Hypoglycemia, H.E.L.P., The Institute for Body Chemistry (215) 525-1225, 9am-9pm, P.O. Box 1338, Bryn Mawr, PA 19010. Offers information on hypoglycemia, counseling, how to start support groups, books on low blood sugar.

Ileitis and Colitis, National Foundation for 800-343-3637. Provides educational materials and refers to local support groups and physicians.

Impotence Information Center 800-843-4315, 24 hours. Provides free information to perspective patients regarding the causes and treatment for impotence.

Incontinence, Simon Foundation for 800-237-4666. Information and publications on incontinence (urine leakage). Free catalog of products. Quarterly newsletter.

Kidney Foundation, National 800-622-9010. Informational materials regarding kidney disorders and organ donations. Local support groups.

Kidney Fund, American 800-638-8299. Grants financial assistance to kidney patients who are unable to pay treatment-related costs. Offers information on organ donations and kidney-related diseases.

La Leche League International 800-525-3243, 9am-3pm, CT. Support to expectant mothers who want to breast feed and mothers who are breast feeding. Educational materials available.

Lamaze 800-368-4404. Offers lists of local certified childbirth educators.

Leukemia Society of America Call 800-555-1212 to request your area's free 800 number. Provides financial aid for patients and sponsors support groups.

Liver Foundation, American 800-223-0179. Provides information, including fact sheets, refers to physicians and support groups. Brochure available on request.

Living Bank 800-528-2971, 24 hours. Registry and referral service for people wanting to donate their tissues, bones, or vital organs to transplantation or research.

Low Blood Sugar See Hypoglycemia

Lung Line/National Asthma Center 800-222-5864. Registered nurses answer questions about asthma, emphysema, chronic bronchitis, allergies, juvenile rheumatoid arthritis, smoking and other respiratory and immune system disorders.

Lupus Foundation of America 800-558-0121. 24 hour recording for callers to leave their names and addresses to receive information. Refers to local affiliates.

Lupus Society, American 800-331-1802. Provides 24 hour recording for callers to leave their names and addresses to receive information on services provided.

Marrow Donor Program, National 800-627-7692. Recruitment of donor types and central registry of donors for any type of fatal blood disease.

HEALTH IS THE ONLY WEALTH

Medic Alert Foundation 800-432-5378. Provides personal medical information for people who cannot speak (unconscious, etc.) for themselves by means of a unique member number on a Medic Alert bracelet or necklace.

Mental Health Association, National 800-969-6642. Makes referrals to mental health groups. Educational brochures

Multiple Sclerosis Society, National 800-532-7667, 24 hour recording for callers to request information and to leave name and address.

Myasthenia Gravis Foundation 800-541-5454, 8:45am-4:45pm CT. Information on services for myasthenia patients. Has low cost prescription services. Local chapters.

Osteoporosis Foundation, National 800-223-9994. Provides literature enabling you to have an indepth understanding of the condition and its ramifications.

Parkinson Disease, American 800-223-2732, 24 hours. Provides information and referrals to patients and families.

Parkinson Foundation, National 800-327-4545, 24 hours. Nurses answer questions about the condition. Makes referrals and provides written materials.

PMS Access 800-222-4767 24 hours. Provides literature and counseling on premenstrual syndrome. Offers referrals to physicians and support groups in caller's area. Publishes Women's Health Access Newsletter.

Rare Disorders, National Organization for 800-999-6673. Offers information on rare disorders listing causes, symptoms, therapy, current research, other sources of information and networking programs.

Reye's Syndrome Foundation, National 800-233-7393. Offers guidance and counseling and awareness materials to public and medical community.

Sexually Transmitted Diseases (STD) Hotline 800-227-8922. Information on STD and confidential referrals for diagnosis and treatment to local clinics offering low-cost or free examinations and treatment.

Sickle Cell Disease, National Association for 800-421-8453, 10am-5pm PT. Offers genetic counseling and an information packet

Spina Bifida Information and Referral 800-621-3141, 24 hours. Provides information and referrals to local chapters.

Spinal Cord Injury Association 800-962-9629, 24 hours. Provides peer counseling to those suffering spinal cord injuries and makes referrals to local chapters and other organizations. Has National Resources Directory and quarterly publication which deals with topics helpful to persons with disabilities.

Spinal Cord Injury Hotline, APA 800-526-3456, 24 hours. Offers literature on spinal cord injuries and makes referrals to organizations and support groups.

Sprue. See Celiac organizations and Gluten Intolerance group.

Stroke Association, National 800-367-1990. Information on referrals, preventions, treatment and rehabilitation to stroke survivors, families and health care providers.

Stroke Network, Courage 800-553-6321, 24 hours. Provides information to stroke patients and receives catalog orders for products for exercise tapes and equipment.

Sudden Infant Death Syndrome Alliance (SIDS) 800-221-7437. Assists bereaved parents; works with families in caring for infants at high risk due to cardiac/respiratory problems. Referrals and support groups. Literature for expectant and new parents.

Sudden Infant Death Syndrome Institute, American 800-232-7437. Answers inquires from families and physicians, phone counseling, literature. Support for families who have suffered a SIDS loss.

Surgery - Second Opinion for Surgery Program Hotline, National 800-638-6833, 8am-8pm, M to F. A medicare hotline.

Thyroid Foundation of America 800-832-8321 Education and support for patients and professionals. Newsletter and literature supplied.

Urologic Disease, American Foundation for 800-242-2383 Education materials and information on research. Prostate cancer support groups.

Visually Impaired, National Association for Parents of 800-562-6265, 24 hours. Provides support and information to parents of visually impaired and multihandicapped individuals. Support groups.

Women's Health America, Inc. 608-833-9102, P.O. Box 9690, Madison, WI, 53715. Provides current, accurate health information to help women make sound consumer decisions concerning their health care and that of their families. Offers quality products and contributes a portion of revenues to support women's health research and education. Free catalog available.

MISCELLANEOUS 800 NUMBERS

MEDICAL

Airlift, Mercy Medical(emergency) 800-296-1217. Provides long distance air ambulance service to patients whose physicians prescribe recovery or special treatment at distant locations.

Aging, National Council on 800-424-9046. Information and publications on various topics, including family caregivers, senior employment and long-term care.

Drinking Water Hotline, Safe 800-426-4791. Information for home water testing, public water regulations and brochures on home water equipment.

Food Safety; Meat and Poultry Hotline 800-535-4555, 10am-4pm ET. Offers safety tips on handling, preparing and storing meat, poultry and eggs. Also supplies free information on label reading.

Hospital Free Care, Hill-Burton 800-638-0742. Information on hospitals and other health facilities participating in the Hill-Burton Free Care Program.

HEALTH IS THE ONLY WEALTH

Medical Libraries near you open to the public 800-338-7657. Refers to medical library near you that is open to the public.

Medicare Telephone Hotline 800-638-6833, 8am-8pm ET. Information on medigap insurance and policies, second opinions and other subjects.

Poison Control Center Check your local phone directory for the poison control center in your area. Information on antidotes to various poisons.

SOCIAL SERVICES

AAA HELP Super Number 800-3A-HELP. Call to get assistance when having car problems while on the road.

Department of Health & Human Services Inspector General's Hotline 800-368-5779 Assists people who have been overbilled or billed for services not rendered. Treats complaints on fraud, waste and abuse of Social Security, Medicare and Medicaid.

FBI - Federal Bureau of Investigation 202-324-2000, 10th & Pennsylvania Ave. NW, Washington, DC 20535.

MADD - Mothers Against Drunk Drivers 800-GET-MADD; National Office, 214-744-6233. Answers questions and sends out general information; Victims Services Department; Public Policy Department on how to change the laws.

Missing Children, National Hotline for 800-843-5678. Hotline for reporting missing children and sightings of missing children. Assistance to law enforcement agents.

IRS for TDD Users 800-4059 TDD, 1/1 to 4/15, 8am-6:45pm; 800-829-1040 Voice, 4/16 to 12/31, 8am-4:30pm. Answers questions on Fed. income tax; medical deductions for telecommunications devices for the deaf (TDD), hearing aids, trained hearing-ear dog; and questions about sending deaf children to special schools.

IRS Inspection Hotline 800-366-4484. Call if you are suspicious about an IRS representative or transaction. When dealing with anyone who claims to be an IRS representative, remember, the IRS generally notifies you by mail.

Retarded Citizens, Association for ARC 817-261-6003, 500 E. Border St., Suite 300, Arlington, TX, 76010. Answers questions and provides referrals to local chapters and support groups. Offers information on publications available from the association.

Runaway Hotline 800-231-6946. Counseling and support for runaways and those thinking about it. Provides runaways with referrals to shelters and temporary place to stay. Offers message relay for children and parents to leave messages for each other. Free ride home.

Runaway Switchboard, National 800-621-4000. Provides crisis intervention and traveler's assistance to runaways. Referrals to shelters nationwide, relays messages to, or sets up conference calls with parent at request of child. Free ride home.

Social Security 800-772-1213; TDD, 800-325-0778. Provides information on all aspects of social security.

PREFACE

By Kathy A. Detweiler, M.A., R.D.

Kathy A. Detweiler is a registered dietitian with a Master's degree in Nutrition Education. She is a member of the American Dietetic Association, Pennsylvania and Philadelphia Dietetic Associations, and Society for Nutrition Education. Currently she is in private practice, counseling patients on an individual basis and consulting for long-term care facilities.

It is refreshing to find a book with the single purpose of presenting health facts. There are no gimmicks, no hidden agendas, no products to sell. The information is given to provide a basis for an individual to make intelligent decisions about their health.

The Krimmels don't tell you what to do, but provide knowledge about nutrition and health that every person can use to modify their diet and to enhance their health status in ways that are appropriate for them. So often we are told what to do and everyone can improve his/her health immediately, as if passing under a magic wand. In reality, everyone is an individual and the choices that we make for our health are just that --- individual choices.

This book is meant to be a wealth of information to further educate ourselves so we can take care of ourselves. From a straight forward explanation of the nutrients we need for healthy cells, to the foods composition table which concludes the book, the information is concise, useful and health-ful.

The Health Information 800 Hotlines in the book are an avenue in themselves to more help and support, especially for those with a specific health problem. The easier it is to reach out for help the more likely one is to do so. Calling an 800 number surely is easy, convenient and inexpensive.

The authors list the basic nutrients with their purposes and continue with the simple truth of weight control with an interesting activity for estimating how many calories you need daily. Vitamins and minerals are described in detail with their functions, sources and related deficiencies. Guidance for the decision to take supplements is provided. The importance of fiber and the types of fiber are clarified. Water is sometimes the forgotten nutrient, but not here. The many functions of water are explained and it is clear why our cells require this nutrient.

A very important skill, I believe, is being able to calculate the percent of calories from fat in a food. This concept is thoroughly explained. The calculation is very easily made although some people don't believe this until they have repeatedly used the equation to become familiar with it and can then use it with ease.

The composition of foods table clearly tells you the calorie content and grams of fat in each food. Browse through the foods table, become familiar with it and keep it handy for looking up foods. As you gradually increase your knowledge of what your diet consists of and how you might like to change your diet, it will become easier to make the choices for yourself!

The journey toward good health should not be a chancy experience. You need reliable information! The Vital Health Facts can be an essential contribution to your health-ful journey.

Kathy A. Detweiler, M.A., R.D.

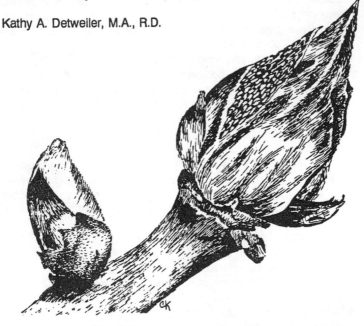

New Life

Charles A. Krimmel

UNDERSTANDING
THE COMPOSITION OF FOODS

Why is it beneficial to know and understand the composition of the foods we eat? Because the components (nutrients), [protein, carbohydrate, fat, fiber, vitamins and minerals] that make up foods are utilized by the cells in the body for specific purposes to keep the cells in your body healthy. If the cells in your body are healthy, you look better, feel better, are happier, and more productive and creative in all aspects of your life. Your relationships (work, social, school & family) are better, you get higher grades, you do more and better work, and it goes on and on and on every day of your life.

Remember, each cell in your body is a power plant. The nutrients from the food you eat are what your cells (power plants) use as fuel to produce the energy for maintaining your life. If you are not getting enough energy from the foods you eat to run your cells efficiently, the systems in your body are not going to function effectively, including your brain and heart.

NUTRIENTS AND THEIR PURPOSES

Proteins - found mostly in dairy products, meat, fowl, fish, eggs, grain and nuts. Comprised of amino acids which are used for the building and repair of the body's tissues (cells).

Carbohydrates - sugars and starches found in fruits and vegetables. There are simple and complex carbohydrates. Simple carbohydrates are those high in natural sugar such as fruits. Complex carbohydrates are foods comprised mainly of starch such as vegetables, grains, nuts and seeds.   Used for energy to perform all body functions and muscular activity. Also help regulate fat and protein metabolism.

Fats - butter, margarine, vegetable oil spreads and vegetables oils. Produces more energy than carbohydrates and are carriers for fat soluble vitamins, A, D, E, and K. Fats slow the stomach's secretion of hydrochloric acid which increase the time needed for digestion, thereby giving a longer period of satisfaction after a meal.   Also needed for steroid production.

Fiber - found in fruits and vegetables. Non soluble fiber helps move "waste" through the digestive tract more rapidly. Soluble fiber decreases fat absorption and helps lower cholesterol levels; slows sugar absorption which is helpful to diabetics and hypoglycemics.

Vitamins - organic substances found in plant and animal tissues and are needed for body maintenance and transforming food into energy. They are generally classified as being water soluble or fat soluble. The water soluble vitamins are usually measured in milligrams and are not stored in the body, the excess is excreted in the urine. The fat soluble vitamins (A, D, E, K) are measured in "International Units" (IU). These vitamins are stored in the body and therefore you must be more careful than with water soluble vitamins not to take too large an amount which may build-up to a toxic level.

Minerals - inorganic substances that have been formed in the earth by nature (iron, copper, calcium, zinc etc.) and have two general body functions, building and regulating. They are found in your bones, blood, muscle, tissue, teeth and nerve cells. Their regulating of functions include such systems as the heart beat, blood clotting, maintenance of the internal pressure of body fluids, nerve responses and transport of oxygen from the lungs to the tissues.

Proteins, carbohydrates and fats are measured (weighed) in grams and each gram has so many calories. Each gram of protein and carbohydrate has 4 calories while each gram of fat has 9 calories, a little over twice that of protein and carbohydrate. This is helpful to know when "counting calories".

Our body needs all of the nutrients and since they are contained in various foods in varying quantities, it is important to eat a wide variety of foods.

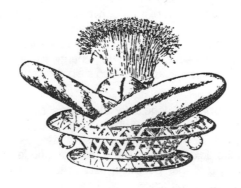

EATING THE PROPER AMOUNT OF CALORIES - WEIGHT CONTROL

To have sufficient energy to function on an efficient level, you must eat enough food to supply your cells with the calories (energy) they need. If for any reason you are eating less fats, sweets, and starches than in the past, you probably should increase your intake of vegetables, legumes, grains, nuts, seeds, fruits, fish, poultry, meats and low fat dairy products in order to get sufficient calories.

REASONS TO BE INTERESTED IN DAILY CALORIE INTAKE

1. To be certain you are eating the appropriate amount of calories (energy) your cells require each day for your activity level.

2. Weight management
   * if you eat more calories than your cells use (burn), the extra calories are converted to fat and stored, resulting in weight gain.
   * if you don't eat enough calories to supply the energy needed, you lose weight by burning up stored fat which is converted to glucose for your cells to use for energy.

3. General health and well being

Some people who suffer from body chemistry conditions get many of their symptoms under control by changing what they eat but still feel tired and worn out at times. Possibly it's because they are not eating sufficient calories for the amount of energy they are expending. For example, would you try to drive 100 miles on one gallon of gas if you have a car, not a motorcycle? Of course not! So don't try to run the cells in your body without sufficient fuel (calories).

DETERMINE THE AMOUNT OF CALORIES YOU SHOULD EAT DAILY

1. Read and follow the directions on the "Nomogram to Estimate Calories Needed" to estimate how many calories you need daily for your age, height, weight and activity. You'll find it interesting and fun to do.

15

2. List all the foods you eat for 7 consecutive days. Use the Nutritive Value of Foods Table to determine the calories in the foods you list.

3. At the end of 7 days, add up the total calories and divide by 7 to give the average amount of calories you had each day.

The objective is to determine the amount of calories you need daily for the energy you expend daily. Much of this process is a crude calculation. If you want to be more accurate, you can use a scale for weighing food, ruler and measuring cups and spoons for measuring portion sizes.

If you do everything correctly, you will have an idea if you are eating sufficient, too few or too many calories for your daily needs. Remember, extra calories are stored as fat.

KEY CONCEPT OF WEIGHT MANAGEMENT

* 3500 calories are equivalent to gaining or losing one pound per week.
* to lose 1 pound, burn up in exercise or eat 3500 calories less per week - best to eat less and exercise to meet 3500 calories.
* to gain 1 pound, eat 3500 calories more per week and/or exercise less.
* 500 calories per day will do just fine, 500 calories x 7 days = 3500 calories per week

HEALTH TIP

Laughter - The Best Medicine

A study at Duke University found that laughter may help prevent heart attacks by defusing anger and lessening stress.

Another study shows that people who use humor as a coping device in everyday life have higher levels of infection-fighting antibodies. Dr. Kathleen Dillon believes, "The benefits of laughter may be cumulative like the benefits of exercise.

If you are not getting enough laughter in your life, change what you are doing.

Have available cartoons, funny movies, humorous books, etc.

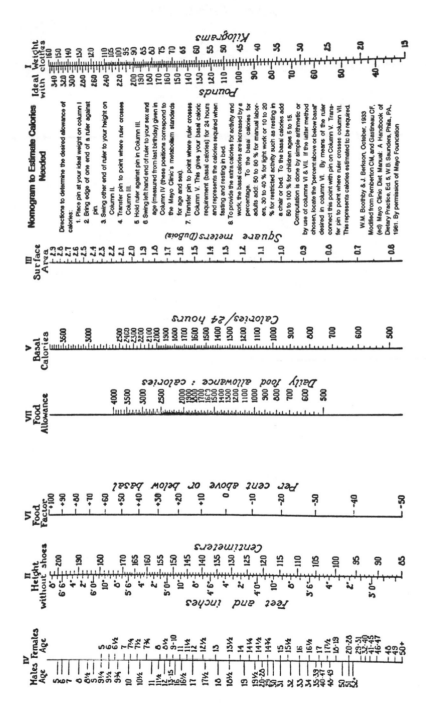

Nomogram to Estimate Calories Needed

Directions to determine the desired allowance of calories:

1. Place pin at your ideal weight on column I
2. Bring edge of one end of a ruler against pin
3. Swing other end of ruler to your height on Column II.
4. Transfer pin to point where ruler crosses Column III.
5. Hold ruler against pin in Column III.
6. Swing left hand end of ruler to your sex and age (measured from last birthday) given in Column IV (these positions correspond to the Mayo Clinic's metabolism standards for age and sex).
7. Transfer pin to point where ruler crosses Column V. This gives your basal caloric requirement (basal calories) for 24 hours and represents the calories required when fasting and resting in bed.
8. To provide the extra calories for activity and work, the basal calories are increased by a percentage. To the basal calories for adults add: 50 to 60 % for manual laborers, 30 to 40 % for light work or 10 to 20 % for restricted activity such as resting in a chair or bed. To the basal calories add 50 to 100 % for children ages 5 to 15.

Computation is done by simple arithmetic or by use of columns VI & VII. If the latter method chosen, locate the "percent above or below basal" desired in column VI. By means of the ruler connect this point with pin on Column V. Transfer pin to point where ruler crosses column VII. This represents calories estimated to be required.

W.M. Boothby & J. Berkson, October, 1933
Modified from Pemberton CM, and Gastineau CF, (ed) Mayo Clinic Diet Manual: A Handbook of Dietary Practice, Ed 5, W.B. Saunders, Phila, PA, 1981. By permission of Mayo Foundation

NOTES

VITAMIN AND MINERAL DEFICIENCIES, RELATED HEALTH PROBLEMS

Nutrients (fats, proteins, carbohydrates, vitamins and minerals) work together to keep us healthy and fit. But if only one is missing or low, it can cause slight to serious problems.

HEALTH PROBLEMS RESULTING FROM DEFICIENCIES

Scurvy - In the days of wooden ships and iron men, many British sailors would come down with scurvy on long voyages. They would have swollen and bleeding gums, tenderness of their joints and muscles, scales on their skin, weakness, poor healing of wounds and bruise easily. No one knew why this occurred until Dr. James Lind took an interest and discovered that if citrus fruit was carried on these long voyages scurvy did not occur. Thereafter limes were always provided on these trips and British sailors became known as "Limeys."

It was later discovered that it was the vitamin C in the limes that prevented scurvy. Vitamin C also works to enhance the absorption of iron, and poor iron absorption can led to anemia, which could complicate scurvy.

Beriberi - This is another condition caused by a deficiency of only one vitamin, thiamine (B_1). In infants, beriberi can cause convulsions, respiratory problems and gastrointestinal difficulties. Adults have fatigue, diarrhea, appetite and weight loss, paralysis, wasting of the limbs due to disturbed nerve function, swelling and heart failure. It is found mostly in the Far East because the basic diet consists mainly of polished rice, which does not supply sufficient thiamine. At times it can be found in other countries when a person's need for thiamine increases due to stressful situations such as infections, pregnancy and alcoholism.

Goiter - At one time, goiter, an enlargement of the thyroid gland, was very prevalent in the U.S. until it was discovered one of the causes was too little natural iodine in the diet. Since seafood and soil along the coast are high in iodine, people living in these areas didn't get goiters caused by iodine deficiency. When iodine was added to salt because of a Federal Government requirement, goiters were practically eliminated from the general population.

Pellagra - A condition caused by a deficiency of the B vitamins Thiamine (B_1), Niacin (B_3), and riboflavin seem to be the ones particularly involved. Its symptoms are diarrhea, loss of appetite and weight, reddened and swollen tongue, weakness, depression and anxiety (sometimes diagnosed as a mental condition). Itch dermatitis on the hands and neck may also occur. It can be cured with a diet high in niacin, thiamine, riboflavin, folic acid and B_{12}.

Rickets - This is usually considered a childhood disease caused by a deficiency of vitamin D, calcium and/or phosphorous. The bones of children with rickets become soft and deformities result when the bones try to support weight which they are too soft to do. The bones are soft because they do not retain calcium. Thus children with rickets have bowlegs, knock-knees, protruding breast bone and narrowed rib cage. They may also have tetany and decayed teeth. Vitamin D, calcium and phosphorous work together and if one is missing or deficient it may result in rickets. Vitamin D aids in the absorption and use of calcium and phosphorous. Vitamin C helps the bones retain calcium and phosphorous.

Most of the above health conditions have been arrested in the U.S. but in some quarters of the world they still prevail. How many other health difficulties have their answers lurking in the shadows of medical research?

Marginal vitamin and mineral deficiencies are frequently found in pregnant women, children, the elderly, alcoholics and drug abusers. During pregnancy, the need for vitamins and minerals increases because of the developing fetus and the extra requirement on the mother's systems.

Children often eat highly refined and fast foods which are low in vitamins and minerals. Frequently the elderly eat small portions of food because of finances, loneliness, etc. Alcoholics and drug abusers many times use their money for alcohol and drugs rather than food. The illicit substances they use deplete the vitamin and minerals in their body.

A long time marginal intake of vitamins and minerals may well be associated with the development of degenerative conditions.

Some examples:

low intake of	may lead to
chromium	high blood sugar levels
magnesium	heart attack
calcium	high blood pressure, osteoporosis
vitamin A	poor eyesight
vitamin B_{12}	pernicious anemia
vitamin C	delayed wound healing

SUPPLEMENTS

Supplements are nutrients that are added to our regular food intake to make up for the nutrients that are low in our diet or are needed in larger quantities than usual. Generally speaking, supplements are vitamins and minerals taken in the form of pills, powders or liquid and come in natural or synthetic preparations.

Vitamins are traditionally divided into two categories:

1. **Fat soluble** vitamins (vitamins A, D, E, and K) can be stored in the body. If an excessive amount is taken, toxic levels can accumulate in storage areas such as the liver. Too much of any fat soluble vitamin can lead to potentially dangerous, long-term problems.

2. **Water soluble** vitamins (B-complex, C, Bioflavonoids) are not stored in the body for an extended period of time. Any excess amount will be excreted in the urine and is therefore valueless.

DO WE NEED VITAMIN AND MINERAL SUPPLEMENTS?

The need for taking vitamin and mineral supplements is a highly debated subject. Each individual has different nutrient needs because he/she is different biochemically, due to:

Age	Nutritional status
Heredity	Ability to digest and utilize food
Activities	Environment--pollutants, temperature, etc.
Mental stress	Physical stress--infections, operations, pregnancy, injuries, etc.

Some examples of situations that can interfere with the quantity of various vitamins we have to utilize are:

* Smoking one cigarette can destroy up to 100 mg of Vitamin C.
* Oral contraceptives and some medications can interfere with the availability of Vitamins B_1, B_6, Folic Acid and Vitamin C.
* Drinking alcoholic beverages interferes with the body's ability to provide adequate nutrients, especially Vitamin B.
* Smog reduces the absorption of Vitamin D for those who live in smoggy cities because smog absorbs the sun's ultraviolet rays.

REASONS FOR CONCERN

Often you hear that eating a well-balanced diet supplies all the vitamins and minerals you need. Eating a well-balanced diet may have been sufficient when most people grew their own food and ate it fresh or dried and used the whole grains for flour and cereals, this may not be as true today. Also any minerals that are not present in the soil where the food is being grown will be missing from that food.

Since vitamins and minerals are so plentiful in nature, the more foods you eat in their natural (raw) forms, the more chance you have of getting an adequate supply of all nutrients. Many vitamins and minerals decrease or are lost during storage and when heated to high temperatures. It has been established that if you use a "no water method," steaming or stir frying methods, to cook your vegetables, you will retain many more of the vitamins and minerals. Since the water left after cooking your vegetables contains some of their vitamins and minerals it can be used in gravies, sauces and soups rather than being poured down the drain.

The more refined (processed) a food is, the more vitamins and minerals that are lost. Flour made from the whole grain of wheat is high in protein, B vitamins, fiber and other vitamins and minerals. But when it is refined into white flour the germ (where the nutrients are) and bran are removed to be sold separately or fed to cattle and pigs. After it is refined, it is also bleached, a process which removes more nutrients. Then it is "enriched" by adding some of the removed nutrients. Why not leave the nutrients in the flour and have whole wheat flour?

You get few really fresh foods (after a fruit or vegetable is picked it loses nutrients each day) or unprocessed foods (nutrients lost during processing) and therefore vitamin and mineral supplements are often required to replace those vitamins and minerals lost. Foods begin losing a portion of their nutrients as soon as they are taken from their natural state. So the fresher foods are and the shorter the cooking time, the more nutrients they will retain. Steaming foods helps retain nutrients better than boiling foods. Frozen foods usually have more nutrients than canned foods because frozen foods are usually packaged sooner than canned food. Also, frozen food usually goes through less processing.

Taking supplements is a personal decision. A dietitian/nutritionist or a nutrition-oriented doctor can give you guidance on what to take, but you should make the final decision predicated on how you feel after taking supplements for an extended period. Some supplements help protect you from degenerative conditions and will not necessarily change the way you feel.

The need for supplements does not occur over night. It may take weeks and even months for the need to show up. As the need occurs, the cells continue to function but at a reduced efficiency. Taking supplements does not produce results overnight. Body chemistry repair takes weeks and sometimes months before full benefits are noticed.

VITAMINS AND MINERALS
FUNCTIONS AND SOURCES

Listed below are the primary vitamins and minerals with what their functions are and the foods in which they are found. The 1989 Recommended Dietary Allowance (RDA), established by the Food and Nutrition Board, the National Academy of Sciences, is also included. The RDA is not intended to indicate individual requirements of therapeutic needs, but to serve as a base reference to adequately meet the nutritional needs of most healthy people.

VITAMINS

Vitamin A - necessary for new cell growth and healthy tissues and vision in dim light. Strengthens cell walls, thus providing mucus membranes defense against infections. Promotes growth, strong bones, healthy skin, hair, teeth and gums. RDA: children under 4 = 2000 IU; children over 4 and adults = 2500 to 5000 IU
  Sources - green and yellow vegetables, peaches, apricots, liver, milk and dairy products, eggs and fish liver oil.

B Vitamins

Thiamine (B_1) - required for normal digestion especially carbohydrates, growth, fertility, lactation, normal functioning of nervous system, muscles, and heart functioning. RDA: children under 4 = 0.7mg; children over 4 and adults = .9 to 1.5mg
  Sources - brewer's yeast, whole grain products, legumes, lean pork, beef, liver, eggs, fish.

Riboflavin (B_2) - helps the body utilize carbohydrates, fats and proteins. Necessary for maintenance of healthy skin, hair, nails and vision. RDA: children under 4 = 0.8mg; children over 4 and adults = 1.1 to 1.7mg
  Sources - milk, meats, poultry, fish, whole grains, broccoli, spinach, asparagus.

Niacin (B_3) - vital for the proper functioning of the nervous system, digestive system and for healthy skin. Aids in stabilizing blood sugar and reducing blood cholesterol. RDA; children under 4 = 9mg; children over 4 and adults = 12 to 20mg
 Sources - liver, lean meats, peas, beans, whole wheat products and peanuts.

Pantothenic Acid (B_5) - vital for proper functioning of adrenal glands, and the synthesis of antibodies, important for healthy skin and nerves and aids in the release of energy form carbohydrates, fat and proteins. RDA: children under 4 = 3mg; children over 4 and adults = 4 to 7mg
 Sources - organ meats, chicken, brewer's yeast, egg yolks, whole grains and nuts.

Pyridoxine (B_6) - necessary for the proper absorption of B_{12}, utilization of protein, proper growth and maintenance of body functions. Also needed for the production of antibodies and red blood cells. Helps release glycogen from the liver and muscles to be used for energy. RDA: children under 4 = 1.0mg; children over 4 and adults = 1 to 2mg
 Sources - organ meats, beef, whole grains, brewer's yeast, seeds, cabbage, blackstrap molasses, milk and eggs.

Cobalamin (B_{12}) - necessary for development of red blood cells and the functioning of all cells, particularly in the bone marrow, nervous system and intestines. Involved with protein, fat and carbohydrate metabolism. RDA: children under 4 = .7mcg; children over 4 and adults = 1 to 2 mcg
 Sources - liver, kidney, lean meat, milk, cheese and eggs.

Biotin - important for metabolism of fats, carbohydrates and protein. RDA: children under 4 = 20mcg; children over 4 and adults = 25 to 100mcg
 Sources - egg yolk, beef liver, soy flour, tomatoes, Brewer's yeast, nonwheat cereals and meats.

Folic acid - necessary for the formation of red blood cells and the metabolism and utilization of protein. Important for the production of RNA and DNA and proper brain function. RDA: children under 4 = 50mcg; children over 4 and adults = 75 to 200mcg; women during pregnancy = 400mcg
 Sources - leafy green vegetables, liver, wheat bran, legumes and yeast.

Vitamin C (Ascorbic Acid)- aids in the growth and repair of connective tissue in skin, ligaments and bones and promotes healing of wounds and burns. Necessary in forming red blood cells and preventing hemorrhaging. Essential for formation of adrenalin. Helps fight bacterial infections and decreases the effects of some allergy-producing substances. RDA: children under 4 = 40mg; children over 4 and adults = 45 to 60mg

Sources - citrus fruits, berries, green and leafy vegetables, peppers, melons, broccoli, potatoes, sweet potatoes, yellow vegetables, and tomatoes, (C is easily destroyed by heat).

Vitamin D - aids in the absorption of calcium and phosphorus which are necessary for bone and teeth formation. Necessary for a stable nervous system, normal heart activity and blood clotting. RDA: children, young adults and women during pregnancy = 400 IU; adults over 24 = 200 IU

Sources - fish liver oils, sardines, herring, salmon, tuna, fortified milk and sunshine.

Vitamin E (Alpha Tocopherol) - is an antioxidant and helps to prevent oxygen from destroying other substances. Plays an important part in cellular respiration of muscles, especially the heart and skeletal, aids them in functioning without as much oxygen. Causes dilation of blood vessels which leads to improved blood flow. RDA: children under 11 = 6 to 7mg; children over 11 and adults = 8 to 10mg

Sources - vegetable oils, whole grains, greens, whole raw seeds and nuts, fish, eggs, meats, cereals and soybeans.

Vitamin K - essential for proper blood clotting, normal liver functioning and converting glucose to glycogen for storage. RDA: children under 4 = 15mcg; children over 4 and adults = 20 to 80mcg

Sources - kelp, alfalfa, leafy green vegetables, milk, dairy products, meats, eggs, cereals, fruits and vegetables.

MINERALS

Calcium - aids in building and maintaining bones and teeth, vital for healthy blood and helps regulate the heartbeat. Assists in blood clotting, muscle growth and contractions, and nerve transmission. RDA: children under 4 = 400 to 800mg; children over 4 and adults = 800 to 1200mg

Sources - milk and dairy products, sardines and almonds.

Chromium - essential component of the organic complex glucose tolerance factor (GTF). Required for glucose utilization, may increase the effectiveness of insulin. May help lower serum cholesterol levels. Safe & adequate intake: children under 4 = 20 to 80mcg; adolescents 30 to 200mcg; adults = 50 to 200mcg

Sources - whole grain breads and cereals, brewer's yeast, lean meats and cheese.

Cobalt - part of vitamin B_{12}. Necessary for normal functioning and maintenance of red blood cells. No RDA
Sources - organ and muscle meats, oysters, clams, and milk.

Copper - involved in the storage and release of iron to form hemoglobin for red blood cells. Involved in protein metabolism and healing. Necessary for proper bone formation and maintenance. Necessary for utilization of Vitamin C. RDA: children under 4 = 0.7 to 1mg; children over 4 and adults = 1 to 3mg
Sources - beef liver, seafood, whole grain products, nuts, seeds and legumes.

Iodine - necessary for the synthesis of the thyroid hormone thyroxin which regulates the rate at which the body uses energy from food and thus is an important regulator of body weight. RDA: children under 4 = 70mcg; children over 4 and adults = 90 to 150mcg
Sources - seafoods, kelp, and iodized salt.

Iron - combines with protein and copper in making hemoglobin; increases resistance to stress and infection, necessary for transporting oxygen and its utilization. Needed for use of B vitamins. RDA: children under 4 = 10mg; children over 4 and adults = 10 to 15mg
Sources - liver, heart, tongue, lean meat, oysters, egg yolk, dark green vegetables, dried fruits and legumes.

Magnesium - activates enzymes necessary for metabolism of carbohydrates and protein, aids in absorption and metabolism of other minerals. Aids in bone growth and is essential for nerves and muscles to function properly. Used in the conversion of blood sugar to energy. RDA; children under 4 = 60 to 80mg; children over 4 and adults = 120 to 350mg
Sources - fresh green vegetables, raw wheat germ, whole grains, seeds, nuts, and bananas.

Manganese - activates enzymes necessary for the body's use of Biotin, B_1, and vitamin C. Necessary for normal skeletal development and for nourishment of the brain and nerves and for proper digestion and utilization of food. Safe & Adequate intake: children under 4 = .5 to 1.5mg children over 4 and adults = 1.5 to 5mg
Sources - whole grain cereals, green vegetables, egg yolks, nuts, seeds and legumes.

Molybdenum - part of two enzymes which are necessary for the transport of iron from the liver and the oxidation of fats. Safe & Adequate intake: children under 11 = 25 to 150mcg; children over 11 and adults = 75 to 250mcg
Sources - dark green leafy vegetables, legumes, milk, organ meats and whole grain cereals.

Phosphorus - aids in most chemical reactions in the body, important for growth, maintenance and repair of cells. Stimulates muscle contractions, including the heart muscle. Needed for normal bone and tooth structure, kidney functioning and transfer of nerve impulses. RDA: children under 4 = 800mg; children over 4 and adults = 800 to 1200mg
Sources - milk, cheese, meat, eggs yolk, whole grains, legumes and nuts.

Potassium - helps regulate body fluid balance and volume, necessary for growth, normal muscle tone and heart action. Aids in converting glucose to glycogen. Estimated minimum requirements: children 1 to 9 = 1,000 to 1600mg; children over 10 and adults = 2000mg
Sources - all vegetables, oranges, bananas, prunes, potatoes and whole grains.

Selenium - antioxidant which may help preserve elasticity of tissues. Helps ensure adequate oxygen supply to certain cells including the heart. Works with vitamin E in metabolism, normal growth and fertility. RDA: children under 4 = 20mcg; children over 4 and adults = 20 to 70mcg
Sources - seafood, kidney, liver, meats, and whole grains.

Sodium - works with potassium to regulate body fluid balance, muscle contraction and expansion, and nerve stimulation. Also aids in keeping blood minerals soluble. Estimated minimum requirements: children 1 to 9 = 225 to 400mg; children over 10 and adults = 500mg
Sources - salt, milk, meat, eggs, baking soda and powder, carrots, beets, spinach and celery.

Sulfur - necessary for good skin, hair and nails; works with other substances for carbohydrate metabolism and strong healthy nerves. Adequate amount supplied when eating sufficient protein.
Sources - meat, eggs, cheese, milk, nuts and legumes

Zinc - necessary for normal absorption, actions of vitamins and growth. Has normalizing effect on the prostate and important in development of reproductive organs. Aids in digestion and metabolism, important in wound and burn healing. RDA: children 10mg; adolescents & adults = 12 to 15mg

27

Sources - whole grain products, legumes, meat, seafood, eggs, and milk.

OTHER NUTRIENTS

Bioflavonoids (citrin, hesperidin, rutin, flavones and flavonals) - may be necessary for the proper absorption and use of vitamin C. Possibility they increase the strength of capillaries and regulate their permeability which helps build protection against infections. No RDA
Sources - white segments of citrus fruits, grapes, plums, black currants, apricots, buckwheat, cherries, blackberries and rose hips.

Choline - aids in utilization of fats and cholesterol. Essential for the health of the liver, kidneys and nerve fibers. No RDA
Sources - egg yolk, liver, brewer's yeast and wheat germ, brain, heart, peanuts and peas.

Essential fatty acids - Linoleic, Linolenic, & Arachidonic - important for tissue strength, cholesterol metabolism, muscle tone, blood clotting and heart action. NO RDA
Sources - wheat germ, nuts, and vegetable oils.

Inositol - may help in metabolism of fats reducing blood cholesterol; needed for growth and survival of cells in bone marrow, eye membranes and intestines. No RDA
Sources - dried lima beans, grapefruit, brewer's yeast, beef heart and brains, peanuts, cabbage and liver.

References: Basic Nutrition and Diet Therapy, ninth edition, 1992; Sue Rodwell Williams, Ph. D., M.P.H., R.D.; Mosby-Year Book, Inc.
The Essential Guide to Vitamins & Minerals, 1992; Elizabeth Somer, M.A., R.D.; Harper Collins Publishers

HEALTH TIP
Prevent Falls
Approximately 9,000 people die each year from falls or related injuries.

Check your home for hazards that could cause a fall - throw rugs, items on stairs, dark halls or stairways, etc.

Store items so you can reach them without standing on a stool or chair.

Slip-proof your tubs and showers. Have non-skid mat next to tub.

Have handrails at all stairs, inside and outside.

THE IMPORTANCE OF FIBER

Dietary fiber is a complex mixture of plant materials. Humans have no enzymes to digest this material and hence fiber has no nutrient value. However, fiber is found to have a relation to good health and disease prevention.

There are two types of fiber:

1. **Insoluble fiber** is composed of:

    cellulose ....stems and leaves of vegetables, skins of fruits and vegetables

    hemicellulose...part of the cell wall of plants; able to absorb water

    lignin.................woody part of plants

2. **Soluble fiber** is composed of:

    gums...............secretions of plants; prevents rapid absorption of glucose in small intestine, slows emptying of stomach, helps in treatment of high cholesterol

    mucilages........plant secretions, seeds, algae and seaweed

    pectins.............intercellular plant material of fruits; can lower amount of fat body absorbs

WHY DO WE NEED FIBER?

Fiber is particularly important for:
* the proper functioning and health of the gastrointestinal tract
* reducing risk of colon and rectal cancer by permitting cancer causing agents in food to pass more quickly through the intestinal tract
* helping regulate blood glucose levels in diabetes
* helping prevent and treat cardiovascular disease
* helping prevent and treat diverticulosis, constipation and hemorrhoids.

Insoluble fiber:
* adds bulk to the remains of the digested food helping to move it through the digestive tract.
* stimulates normal muscle action of the intestines which promotes

normal elimination and hastens the passage of the stool through the colon.
* helps to satisfy appetite by creating a full feeling.

Soluble fiber:
* has cholesterol lowering effect; helpful in preventing and treating cardiovascular disease.
* slows glucose absorption; helpful for diabetics and low blood sugar sufferers.
* absorbs water forming a large bulk which slows foods from leaving the stomach.
* provides fermentation material for important colon bacteria to grow on.

HOW MUCH FIBER IS NEEDED DAILY?

According to national surveys, individuals eat between 10 and 17 grams of fiber daily. There is no RDA standard for dietary fiber but a high fiber diet is associated with a reduced risk for colon cancer, cardiovascular disease, diabetes, hypertension and several intestinal disorders. The National Cancer Institute recommends 25 to 35 grams of fiber daily.

It is best to gradually increase your fiber intake since a sudden increase in fiber can lead to intestinal cramps, bloating and gas.

HOW TO GET ADEQUATE FIBER

All vegetables, fruits and whole grains have dietary fiber. Animal products have no dietary fiber. Eating a variety of vegetables, fruits and whole grain products is the best way to get adequate fiber. Cooking can reduce the fiber content of foods so use the shortest cooking time possible. When possible, eat vegetables and fruits with their skins. Use whole grain flours for baking; eat whole grain cereals, breads and other grain dishes. Increase the amount of dried beans and peas and nuts you eat.

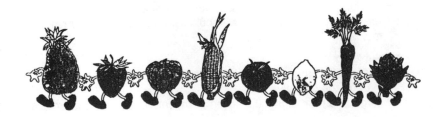

FIBER CONTENT OF SOME FOODS*

Foods	Serving	Total Fiber(gms)	Soluble Fiber(gms)	Insoluble Fiber(gms)
BREADS & CEREALS				
Bran Cereal(100%)	½ cup	10.0	0.3	9.7
Popcorn	3 cups	2.8	0.8	2.0
Rye bread	1 slice	2.7	0.8	1.9
Whole grain bread	1 slice	2.7	0.08	2.8
Rye wafers	3	2.3	0.06	2.2
Corn grits	½ cup ck.	1.9	0.6	1.3
Oatmeal	½ cup ck.	1.6	0.5	1.1
Graham cracker	2	1.4	0.04	1.4
Brown rice	½ cup ck.	1.3	0	1.3
French bread	1 slice	1.0	0.4	0.6
Dinner roll	1	0.8	0.03	0.8
Egg noodles	½ cup ck.	0.8	0.3	0.8
Spaghetti	½ cup ck.	0.8	0.02	0.8
White bread	1 slice	0.8	0.03	0.8
White rice	½ cup ck.	0.5	0	0.5
FRUITS (raw)				
Apple	1 small	3.9	2.3	1.6
Blackberries	½ cup	3.7	0.7	3.0
Pear	1 small	2.5	0.6	1.9
Strawberries	3/4 cup	2.4	0.9	1.5
Plums	2 med.	2.3	1.3	1.0
Tangerine	1 med	1.6	1.4	0.4
Apricots	2 med	1.3	0.9	0.4
Banana	1 small	1.3	0.6	0.7
Grapefruit	1/2	1.3	0.9	0.4
Peaches	1 med.	1.0	0.5	0.5
Cherries	10	0.9	0.3	0.6
Pineapple	1/2 cup	0.8	0.2	0.6
Grapes	10	0.4	0.1	0.3
LEGUMES				
Kidney beans	½ cup	4.5	0.5	4.0
White beans	½ cup	4.2	0.4	3.8
Pinto beans	½ cup	3.0	0.3	2.7
Lima beans	½ cup	1.4	0.2	1.2
NUTS				
Almonds	10	1.0	n/a	n/a
Peanuts	10	1.0	n/a	n/a
Black walnuts	1 tsp.	0.6	n/a	n/a
Pecans	2	0.5	n/a	n/a
VEGETABLES (cooked)				
Peas	½ cup	5.2	2.0	3.2
Parsnips	½ cup	4.4	.04	4.0
Potatoes	1 small	3.8	2.2	1.6
Broccoli	½ cup	2.6	1.6	1.0
Zucchini	½ cup	2.5	1.1	1.4
Summer squash	½ cup	2.3	1.1	1.2
Lettuce(raw)	½ cup	0.5	0.2	0.3

*The Nutrition Desk Reference

WATER, AN
ULTIMATE SUBSTANCE

Water, water is everywhere and most people still aren't drinking enough! Although water has no calories, it is as important to drink 6 to 8 eight ounce glasses of water a day as it is to eat the proper amount of calories. Did you know oxygen is the only substance more important to the body than water? Water is the most abundant nutrient in our body (about 2/3 of body weight) and is vital to human existence. The cells in your body require moisture to be healthy.

Ways in which water is important in nearly every body process:

* circulates through the body in the blood, body secretions and tissue fluids helping to carry nutrients and other substances to all the cells in the body to help meet their needs for proper functioning.
* necessary for all building functions in the body and digestion, absorption, circulation, and excretion.
* necessary for maintaining a stable body temperature. When your temperature rises, sweat is produced, evaporates and cools the body.
* essential for carrying waste material out of the body and helps form a soft stool which aids in preventing constipation and assists in the avoidance of painful hemorrhoids.

Through excretion and perspiration the average adult loses about 3 quarts of water daily. The amount lost is related to activity, temperature, functional losses (diarrhea, vomiting, etc.), metabolic needs and age.

Nearly all foods, especially fruits and vegetables, contain water that is absorbed by the body during digestion.

Drinking beverages with some water in them doesn't mean you are getting sufficient water. Caffeine in sodas, coffee, tea, etc. acts as a diuretic. You may notice that after drinking beverages with caffeine, that you go to the bathroom more frequently. That is caused by caffeine, not just that you drank something. Therefore, the more caffeine you have, the more water you should drink to replace what is lost as a result of the diuretic effect of caffeine.

The elderly have a tendency to lose their desire for water and need to be reminded to drink sufficient water.

THE SATURATED FAT
AND
CHOLESTEROL CONNECTION

The typical American gets about 35% to 40% of his/her calories from fat. The American Heart Association and cholesterol experts strongly recommend that you should get no more than 20% to 30% of your total daily calories from fat.

There are two major categories of dietary fat:
1. Saturated fat
2. Unsaturated fat - comprised of two types of fat
   polyunsaturated fat
   monounsaturated fat

All foods containing fat are comprised of a mixture of the above fats. The combination of these fats in the foods you eat make up the total amount of fat you eat daily.

The most effective way to lower your cholesterol is to eat less saturated fat. It is very important that no more than 5% to 10% of your total calories come from saturated fat because research has established; **it is saturated fat that raises blood cholesterol more than anything else you eat, even more than the cholesterol you eat.**

Reasons for eating less fat:
* To make it easier to reduce saturated fat intake
* To promote weight control

The major sources of saturated fats are:
* Animal products (meats, whole milk and its products)
* Three vegetable fats (coconut oil, palm and palm kernel oils & cocoa butter)
* Hydrogenated vegetable oils - act as saturated fats

Because most fats are not able to be seen in products, you must carefully read ingredient lists and nutrition information on packaged foods to determine what the fat content is. Many packages list the oils and/or shortenings in the products, and some may list how many grams of saturated fat there are per serving. Using this information will help you determine which foods are appropriate for you.

By doing some basic math, you can easily determine the number of calories or grams of total fat you should be limiting yourself to daily.

For example: If you eat 1800 calories per day;
* Multiply 1800 by .20 and then .30 (20% & 30%) and you will see that your total calories from fat should be between 360 to 540 calories daily.
* Divide the 360 & 540 calories by 9 (grams of fat per each calorie) to determine the number of grams of fat you may eat, which is a total of 40 to 60 grams of fat daily.

REMEMBER, only 5% to 10% of your total daily calories should come from saturated fat. So do the same math for saturated fat:
* Multiple .05 and .10 (5% & 10%) times 1800 which equals 90 and 180 calories of saturated fat.
* Divide the 90 & 180 calories by 9 which equals 10 to 20 grams of saturated fat daily.
* Subtract the 10 and 20 grams of allowed saturated fat from the 40 - 60 grams of total fat allowed leaving a total of **30 to 40 grams of unsaturated fat and 10 to 20 grams of saturated fat daily.**

ALWAYS REMEMBER, saturated fat raises blood cholesterol more than anything else you eat, even more than the cholesterol you eat.

Since fat is usually listed in grams on the nutrition information area of packaged foods, it is convenient to know your fat allowance in both calories and grams. Some packages are now listing the percentage of fat per serving which is helpful.

When using the nutrition information on packages, you can quickly calculate the percentage of fat per serving by:
* multiplying the grams of fat per serving by 9
* dividing that answer by the calories per serving.

For example, if the nutrition information per serving lists:

Serving size............................... 1 cup
Calories... 240
Fat.. 3 grams

Multiply 3 grams of fat x 9 calories per gram = 27 calories of fat ÷ 240 calories per serving = .059 = 6% fat per serving.
Always check to be certain the serving size is a realistic amount.

The Nutritive Value of Food Table in this book gives you the amount of the different types of fat contained in the various foods you eat.

For a total understanding of cholesterol management, see order form in back of book for the Cholesterol Lowering & Controlling Handbook & Cookbook.

EXERCISE

In America of yesteryear, most people did a very great amount of physical activity to satisfy their daily needs. Subsequently people got exercise from their daily activities. However, these days we have so many labor saving devices and services that there is no longer a need to do much physical activity to fulfill daily needs. Because of the cultural changes, one must now be certain to get physical activity through planned exercise.

Leading a sedentary life while aging can result in an inappropriate decline in stamina, the capacity to do normal physical activity and increase the chance of injury and heart disease. For a healthy body chemistry and overall health and well-being, exercise plays as important a role as food, and in some respects more of one. You should include it in your everyday schedule--just as you include food and water.

WHY EXERCISE?

To help:

keep joints & muscle flexible	strengthen muscles
lose weight (use up calories)	control blood cholesterol levels
Relieve stress	increase oxygen intake and distribution

Oxygen is the most important substance required by the cells in your body. You can live days without food and water but only 5 minutes without oxygen. The amount of oxygen you take in is in direct proportion to the amount of physical activity you do.

Exercise is one of the vital means of building a wall of resistance between you and degenerative conditions. Once you have a degenerative condition, exercise is one of the vital means of overcoming or controlling the condition.

WHAT DOES EXERCISE DO?

Exercise makes us stronger and healthier by improving the oxygen intake and delivery to our body. When we exercise we breathe deeper and faster thereby increasing our lung capacity. Exercise also makes the heart pump (beat) stronger and faster which strengthens the heart muscle. Our major blood vessels enlarge due to the increased rate and amount of blood being pumped through them. All of this leads to an improved ability to use oxygen and an increased ability to deliver nutrients to each and every cell by our improved circulatory system, Improved digestion,

35

absorption, metabolism, and the improved elimination of our waste products.

PHILOSOPHY OF EXERCISE

Exercise is very personal, what is suited to one person may be totally unsuited to another--for a variety of reasons. For starters, you must take a very close look at where you are now in relation to your physical well-being and where you wish to go. After a clear picture is seen of the now and then--you can begin charting a course on how to get there and by what stages. You must decide on the time of day and the type and degree of exercise. Each area of the program must remain interesting to you and goal oriented.

You should not feel you have to do the same activities for exercise every day. If you were on vacation at the seashore in the ocean fighting the waves and briskly walking the beach, that would be your exercise rather than what you normally do for exercise.

Another factor of importance and probably of the highest priority is that you must make sure the exercise program you choose is fun and interesting to you. Avoid fad or cosmetic type exercises and programs. It has been established scientifically that people who participate in exercises and activities that are not pleasurable to them do themselves more harm than good. Regardless of scientific findings, if you were to just sit and ponder the mood that is generated when participating in activities that are not to your liking you will gradually see the point and importance of this issue.

The value of exercise is in direct proportion to how your body's mechanisms are responding to the mood which is being created during the given activity.

Before you begin exercising you should be checked by your doctor to be certain you are physically suited to your planned exercise program.

TYPES OF EXERCISE

Three types of exercise:
1. Warm-up   2. Conditioning   3. Circulatory (aerobic)

Warm-up exercises stretch and limber up the muscles and increase the heart and lung action, thereby preparing the body for greater exertion and reducing the possibility of unnecessary strain. These should be done before any other exercise.

Examples of warm-up exercises:
Bending and stretching   Knee bends
Bending side to side   Knee lifts

Conditioning exercises are to tone up major muscles such as the abdomen, back, legs, arms, etc.

Examples of conditioning exercises:

| Knee push ups | Sit ups | Hiking |
| Touching toes | Bicycling | Skating |

Circulatory exercises (aerobic) are activities that raises your heart rate above its resting point. They should be done for 20 to 30 minutes at least three times per week to stimulate and strengthen the circulatory and respiratory systems.

Examples of circulatory (aerobic) exercises:

| Brisk walking | Bicycling | Swimming |
| Jumping rope | Tennis-singles | Cross-country skiing |

PULSE TAKING

In order for aerobic exercise to be effective and to produce the desired results, your pulse rate must increase to a certain point. Exercise should be done for 20 to 30 minutes at a time, at least three to four times a week. See the chart below for what your pulse rate should increase to during your exercise.

PULSE RATE DURING EXERCISE			
AGE	*PULSE RATE*	*AGE*	*PULSE RATE*
20	120–150 beats per minute	50	102–127 beats per minute
25	117–146 beats per minute	55	99–123 beats per minute
30	114–142 beats per minute	60	96–120 beats per minute
35	111–138 beats per minute	65	93–116 beats per minute
40	108–135 beats per minute	70	90–113 beats per minute
45	105–131 beats per minute		

Source: U.S. Department of Health and Human Services

To take your pulse, put the 3 middle fingers of your right hand on the under side of your left wrist below your thumb. Count the beats for 30 seconds and multiply by 2 for how many beats per minute.

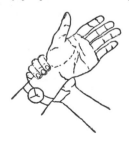

THINGS TO REMEMBER WHEN EXERCISING

When is it most favorable for you to exercise? Some people find that when they first get up in the morning is most suitable.Decide when you feel the best or have nothing pressing to do. For some, the evening is the most ideal time.

* Don't "bankrupt" yourself of your energy reserve--never do more exercise and use more energy than you can afford to spend.

* It is preferable that you wait for at least an hour after you eat before doing any strenuous activity so it doesn't interfere with your digestion.

* If you have not been doing any type of exercise, start out slowly by going for short walks. Gradually increase the briskness and distance.

* When your exercise time becomes more strenuous and longer, have an apple or something else with you to eat in case you feel the need for food.

* Do activities that are enjoyable to you, your activities can change with the seasons--swimming in summer; ice skating or cross country skiing or sledding in the winter; biking or hiking in the fall and spring. Of course brisk walking can be done almost anytime and anywhere. Doing yard or garden work or hard housework (scrubbing) for a couple of hours is also good.

SUMMARY

Exercise should be an activity that you enjoy doing, and is done at least 3 to 4 times a week in pleasing surroundings. Aerobic exercise should increase your pulse rate, improve muscle tone, circulation, digestion, metabolism and elimination as well as help supply sufficient oxygen to each and every cell to help insure efficient functioning. The importance of exercise cannot be overstated.

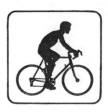

COMPOSITION OF FOODS
NUTRITIVE VALUE OF FOODS TABLE

Listing Calorie, Protein, Carbohydrate, Fat
and Cholesterol Content of Various Foods

FOODS ARE GROUPED
UNDER THE FOLLOWING MAIN HEADINGS

Beverages
Dairy Products
Eggs
Fats & Oils
Fish & Shellfish
Fruit & Fruit Juices
Grain Products
Legumes, Nuts & Seeds

Meat & Meat Products
Mixed Dishes & Fast Foods
Poultry & Poultry Products
Soups, Sauces & Gravies
Sugar & Sweets
Vegetables & Vegetable Products
Miscellaneous

The Nutritive Value of Foods Table is a valuable tool in helping you understand the composition of the foods you are eating.

The Table allows you to determine:
* the amount of calories you are eating
* which foods are low in fat for losing weight
* which foods are low in saturated fat for controlling
  your cholesterol count
* which foods are most beneficial for you

Data in following table from the United States Department of Agriculture, Human Nutrition Information Service;
Home and Garden Bulletin Number 72

| Foods | Approximate Measure | Weight | Calories | Protein | Carbohydrate | Total Fat | Fats | | | Cholesterol |
| | Portion | Grams | Calories | Grams | Grams | Grams | Saturated | Mono-unsaturated | Poly-unsaturated | Milligrams |
							Grams	Grams	Grams	
Beverages										
Alcoholic										
Beer										
Regular	12 oz	360	150	1	13	0	0	0	0	0
Light	12 oz	355	95	1	5	0	0	0	0	0
Gin, rum, vodka, whiskey										
80-proof..........	1½ oz	42	95	0	tr	0	0	0	0	0
86-proof..........	1½ oz	42	105	0	tr	0	0	0	0	0
90-proof..........	1½ oz	42	110	0	tr	0	0	0	0	0
Wines										
Dessert	3½ oz	103	140	tr	8	0	0	0	0	0
Table										
Red	3½ oz	102	75	tr	3	0	0	0	0	0
White	3½ oz	102	80	tr	3	0	0	0	0	0
Carbonated										
Club soda..........	1 oz	30	0	0	0	0	0	0	0	0
Cola type										
Regular..........	1 oz	30	13	3	0	0	0	0	0	0
Diet	1 oz	30	tr	tr	0	0	0	0	0	0
Ginger ale..........	1 oz	30	10	3	0	0	0	0	0	0
Grape..........	1 oz	30	15	4	0	0	0	0	0	0
Lemon-lime..........	1 oz	30	13	3	0	0	0	0	0	0
Orange	1 oz	30	15	4	0	0	0	0	0	0
Pepper type..........	1 oz	30	13	30	0	0	0	0	0	0
Root beer	1 oz	30	13	3	0	0	0	0	0	0

	Grams								
Cocoa & chocolate-flavored									
See dairy products									
Coffee									
Brewed ....6 oz	180	tr	tr	tr	tr	tr	tr	tr	0
Instant, 2 tsp. powder in 6 oz. water ....6 oz	182	tr	tr	1	tr	tr	tr	tr	0
Fruit drinks									
Canned									
Fruit punch drink..........6 oz	190	85	tr	22	tr	0	0	0	0
Grape drink.............6 oz	187	100	tr	26	tr	0	0	0	0
Pineapple-grapefruit juice drink....6 oz	187	90	tr	23	tr	tr	tr	tr	0
Frozen									
Lemonade concentrate									
Undiluted ....6 oz	219	425	tr	112	tr	tr	tr	tr	0
Diluted with 4⅓ parts water by volume ....6 oz	185	80	tr	21	tr	tr	tr	tr	0
Limeade concentrate									
Undiluted ....6 oz	218	410	tr	108	tr	tr	tr	tr	0
Diluted with 4⅓ parts water by volume ....6 oz	185	75	tr	20	tr	tr	tr	tr	0
Fruit juices, see under fruits									
Milk beverages, see dairy products									
Tea									
Brewed ....8 oz	240	tr	tr	tr	tr	tr	tr	tr	0
Instant, powder									
Unsweetened, 1 tsp. powder + 8 oz water.......8 oz	241	tr	tr	1	tr	tr	tr	tr	0
Sweetened, 3 tsp. powder + 8 oz water.......8 oz	262	85	tr	22	tr	tr	tr	tr	0

(tr indicates nutrient present in trace amount)

Dairy Products

Foods	Approximate Measure (Portion)	Weight (Grams)	Calories (Calories)	Protein (Grams)	Carbohydrate (Grams)	Total Fat (Grams)	Fats Saturated (Grams)	Fats Mono-unsaturated (Grams)	Fats Poly-unsaturated (Grams)	Cholesterol (Milligrams)
Butter	½ cup	113	810	1	tr	92	57	26	3.4	247
	1 Tbs	14	100	tr	tr	11	7.1	3.3	0.4	31
	1 pat	5	35	tr	tr	4	2.5	1.2	0.2	11
Cheese										
Natural										
Blue	1 oz	28	100	6	1	8	5.3	2.2	0.2	21
Camembert	1.33 oz	38	115	8	tr	9	5.8	2.7	0.3	27
Cheddar	1 oz	28	115	7	tr	9	6.0	2.7	0.3	30
Cube	1 in	17	70	4	tr	6	3.6	1.6	0.2	18
Shredded	1 cup	113	455	28	1	37	23.8	10.6	1.1	119
Cottage (curd not pressed down)										
Creamed (cottage cheese, 4% fat)										
Large curd	1 cup	225	235	28	6	10	6.4	2.9	0.3	34
Small curd	1 cup	210	215	26	6	9	6.0	2.7	0.3	31
With fruit	1 cup	226	280	22	30	8	4.9	2.2	0.2	108
Lowfat (2%)	1 cup	226	205	31	8	4	2.8	1.2	0.1	19
Uncreamed (cottage cheese dry curd, less than ½% fat)	1 cup	145	125	25	3	1	0.4	0.2	tr	10
Cream	1 oz	28	100	2	1	10	6.2	2.8	0.4	31
Feta	1 oz	28	75	4	1	6	4.2	1.3	0.2	25
Mozzarella, made with:										
Whole milk	1 oz	28	80	6	1	6	3.7	1.9	0.2	22
Part skim milk	1 oz	28	80	8	1	5	3.1	1.4	0.1	15
Muenster	1 oz	28	105	7	tr	9	5.4	2.5	0.2	27

Parmesan, grated:									
Not pressed down .... 1 cup	100	455	42	4	30	19.1	8.7	0.7	79
1 Tbs	5	25	tr	2	1.0	0.4	tr	4	4
Provolone .... 1 oz	28	130	12	1	9	5.4	2.5	0.2	22
1 oz	28	100	7	1	8	4.8	2.1	0.2	20
Ricotta, made with:									
Whole milk. .... 1 cup	246	430	28	7	32	20.4	8.9	0.9	124
Part skim milk. .... 1 cup	246	340	28	13	19	12.1	5.7	0.6	76
Swiss .... 1 oz	28	105	8	1	8	5.0	2.1	0.3	26
Pasteurized process:									
American .... 1 oz	28	105	6	tr	9	5.6	2.5	0.3	27
Swiss .... 1 oz	28	95	7	1	7	4.5	2.0	0.2	24
Pasteurized process cheese food,									
American .... 1 oz	28	95	6	2	7	4.4	2.0	0.2	18
Pasteurized process cheese spread,									
American .... 1 oz	28	80	5	2	6	3.8	1.8	0.2	16
Cream, sweet:									
Half & Half .... 1 cup	242	315	7	10	28	17.3	8.0	1.0	89
1 Tbs	15	20	tr	1	2	1.1	0.5	0.1	6
Light .... 1 cup	240	470	6	9	46	28.8	13.4	1.7	159
1 Tbs	15	30	tr	1	3	1.8	0.8	0.1	10
Whipping, unwhipped:									
Light .... 1 cup	239	700	5	7	74	46.2	21.7	2.1	265
1 Tbs	15	45	tr	tr	5	2.9	1.4	0.1	17
Heavy ... . 1 cup	238	820	5	7	88	54.8	25.4	3.3	326
1 Tbs	15	50	tr	tr	6	3.5	1.6	0.2	21
Whipped topping (pressurized) ..... 1 cup	60	155	2	7	13	8.3	3.9	0.5	46
1 Tbs	3	10	tr	tr	1	0.4	0.2	tr	2
Cream, sour .... 1 cup	230	495	7	10	48	30.0	13.9	1.8	102
1 Tbs	12	25	tr	1	3	1.6	0.7	0.1	5

Dairy Products continued

Cream products, imitation (made with vegetable fat):

Foods	Approximate Measure — Portion	Weight Grams	Calories	Protein Grams	Carbohydrate Grams	Total Fat Grams	Fats			Cholesterol Milligrams
							Saturated Grams	Mono-unsaturated Grams	Poly-unsaturated Grams	
Sweet:										
Creamers:										
Liquid (frozen)	1 Tbs	15	20	tr	2	1	1.4	tr	tr	0
Powdered	1 tsp	2	10	tr	1	1	0.7	tr	tr	0
Whipped topping:										
Frozen	1 cup	75	240	1	17	19	16.3	1.2	0.4	0
	1 Tbs	4	15	tr	1	1	0.9	0.1	tr	0
Powdered, made with whole milk	1 cup	80	150	3	13	10	8.5	0.7	0.2	8
	1 Tbs	4	10	tr	1	tr	0.4	tr	tr	tr
Pressurized	1 cup	70	185	1	11	16	13.2	1.3	0.2	0
	1 Tbs	4	10	tr	1	1	0.8	0.1	tr	0
Sour dressing (filled cream type product, nonbutterfat)	1 cup	235	415	8	11	39	31.2	4.6	1.1	13
	1 Tbs	12	20	tr	1	2	1.6	0.2	0.1	1
Ice cream, vanilla:										
Regular (11% fat):										
Hardened	1 cup	133	270	5	32	14	8.9	4.1	0.5	59
	3 oz	50	100	2	12	5	3.4	1.6	0.2	22
Soft serve (frozen custard)	1 cup	173	375	7	38	23	13.5	6.7	1.0	153
Rich (16% fat), hardened	1 cup	148	350	4	32	24	4.7	6.8	0.9	88

Food	grams								
Ice milk, vanilla:									
Hardened (4% fat)..............1 cup	131	185	5	29	6	3.5	1.6	0.2	18
Soft serve (3% fat) ....1 cup	175	225	8	38	5	2.9	1.3	0.2	13
Sherbet (2% fat) ....1 cup	193	270	2	59	4	2.4	1.1	0.1	14
Milk									
Fluid:									
Whole (3.3% fat)...............1 cup	244	150	8	11	8	5.1	2.4	0.3	33
Lowfat (2%):									
No milk solids added ....1 cup	244	120	8	12	5	2.9	1.4	0.2	18
Milk solids added, label claim									
<10 g protein per cup.......1 cup	245	125	9	12	5	2.9	1.4	0.2	18
Lowfat (1%):									
No milk solids added ....1 cup	244	100	8	12	3	1.6	0.7	0.1	10
Milk solids added, label claim									
<10 g protein per cup.......1 cup	245	105	9	12	2	1.5	0.7	0.1	10
Nonfat (skim):									
No milk solids added ....1 cup	245	85	8	12	tr	0.3	0.1	tr	4
Milk solids added, label claim									
<10 g protein per cup.......1 cup	245	90	9	12	1	0.4	0.2	tr	5
Buttermilk..........................1 cup	245	100	8	12	2	1.3	0.6	0.1	9
Canned:									
Condensed, sweet...............1 cup	306	980	24	166	27	16.8	7.4	1.0	104
Evaporated:									
Whole milk........................1 cup	252	340	17	25	19	11.6	5.9	0.6	74
Skim milk..........................1 cup	255	200	19	29	1	0.3	0.2	tr	9
Dried:									
Buttermilk..........................1 cup	120	465	41	59	7	4.3	2.0	0.3	83
Nonfat, instant:									
Envelope, 3.2 oz.....................1	91	325	32	47	1	0.4	0.2	tr	17
cup....................................1 cup	68	245	24	35	tr	0.3	0.1	tr	12

Dairy Products continued

Foods	Approximate Measure	Weight	Calories	Protein	Carbohydrate	Total Fat	Fats			Cholesterol
							Saturated	Mono-unsaturated	Poly-unsaturated	
	Portion	Grams	Calories	Grams	Grams	Grams	Grams	Grams	Grams	Milligrams
Milk beverages:										
Chocolate milk (comm):										
Regular ....1 cup		250	210	8	26	8	5.3	2.5	0.3	31
Low fat (2%) ....1 cup		250	180	8	26	5	3.1	1.5	0.2	17
Lowfat (1%) ....1 cup		250	160	8	26	3	1.5	0.8	0.1	7
Cocoa & chocolate flavored										
Powder containing nonfat										
dry milk ....1 oz		28	100	3	22	1	0.6	0.3	tr	1
Prepared (6 oz. water										
+ 1 oz. powder)..........1 serv		206	100	3	22	1	0.6	0.3	tr	1
Powder without nonfat										
dry milk ....¾ oz		21	75	1	19	1	0.3	0.2	tr	0
Prepared (8 oz. whole milk										
+ ¾ oz. powder) ....1 serv		265	225	9	30	9	5.4	2.5	0.3	33
Eggnog (commercial)..........1 cup		254	340	10	4	19	11.3	5.7	0.9	149
Malted milk:										
Chocolate:										
Powder .... ¾ oz		21	85	1	18	1	0.5	0.3	0.1	1
Prepared (8 oz. whole milk										
+ ¾ oz. powder) ....1 serv		265	235	9	29	9	5.5	2.7	0.4	34

Natural:									
Powder..............¾ oz	21	85	3	15	2	0.9	0.5	0.3	4
Prepared (8 oz. whole milk + ¾ oz. powder)..........1 serv	265	235	11	27	10	6.0	2.9	0.6	37
Shakes, thick:									
Chocolate.............10 oz	283	335	9	60	8	4.8	2.2	0.3	33
Vanilla...............10 oz	283	315	11	50	9	5.3	2.5	0.3	30
Yogurt:									
With added milk solids:									
Made with lowfat milk.									
Fruit flavored...........8 oz	227	230	10	43	2	1.6	0.7	0.1	10
Plain..................8 oz	227	145	12	16	4	2.3	1.0	0.1	14
Made with nonfat milk.....8 oz	227	125	13	17	tr	0.3	0.1	tr	4
Without added milk solids:									
Made with whole milk......8 oz	227	140	8	11	7	4.8	2.0	0.2	29
Eggs									
Eggs, large:									
Raw:									
Whole..................1 egg	50	80	6	1	6	1.7	2.2	0.7	210
White of egg............1	33	15	3	tr	tr	0.0	0.0	0.0	0
Yolk....................1	17	65	3	tr	6	1.7	2.2	0.7	210
Cooked:									
Fried, in butter.........1 egg	46	95	6	1	7	2.7	2.7	0.8	214
Hard-cooked.............1	50	80	6	1	6	1.7	2.2	0.7	210
Poached................1	50	80	6	1	6	1.7	2.2	0.7	209
Scrambled or omelet, milk added, in butter........1 egg	64	110	7	2	8	3.2	2.9	0.8	218

Fats and Oils

Foods	Approximate Measure (Portion)	Weight (Grams)	Calories (Calories)	Protein (Grams)	Carbohydrate (Grams)	Total Fat (Grams)	Fats Saturated (Grams)	Fats Mono-unsaturated (Grams)	Fats Poly-unsaturated (Grams)	Cholesterol (Milligrams)
Fats, cooking (vegetable shortenings).............	1 cup	205	1,810	0	0	205	51.3	91.2	53.5	0
	1 Tbs	13	115	0	0	13	3.3	5.8	3.4	0
Lard.............	1 cup	205	1,850	0	0	205	80.4	92.5	23.0	195
	1 Tbs	13	115	0	0	13	5.1	5.9	1.5	12
Margarine:										
Imitation, about 40% fat, soft	1 Tbs	14	50	tr	tr	5	1.1	2.2	1.9	0
Regular, about 80% fat:										
Hard:										
stick.............	½ cup	113	810	1	1	91	17.9	40.5	28.7	0
	1 Tbs.	14	100	tr	tr	11	2.2	5.0	3.6	0
1" sq. pat.............	1 pat	5	35	tr	tr	4	0.8	1.8	1.3	0
Soft.............	1 Tbs	14	100	tr	tr	11	1.9	4.0	4.8	0
Spread, about 60% fat:										
Hard:										
Stick.............	½ cup	113	610	1	0	69	15.9	29.4	20.5	0
	1 Tbs	14	75	tr	0	9	2.0	3.6	2.5	0
1" sq. pat.............	1 pat	5	25	tr	0	3	0.7	1.3	0.9	0
Soft.............	1 Tbs	14	75	tr	0	9	1.8	4.4	1.9	0
Oils, salad or cooking:										
Canola.............	1 Tbs	14	125	0	0	14	1.0	9.0	4.0	0
Coconut.............	1 Tbs	14	117	0	0	14	12.0	1.0	0.2	0
Corn.............	1 Tbs	14	125	0	0	14	1.8	3.4	8.2	0

Food	Measure								
Olive	1 Tbs	14	125	0	0	14	1.9	10.3	1.2	0
Palm	1 Tbs	14	120	0	0	14	7.0	5.0	1.0	0
Peanut	1 Tbs	14	125	0	0	14	2.4	6.5	4.5	0
Safflower	1 Tbs	14	125	0	0	14	1.3	1.7	10.4	0
Soybean oil, partially hydrogenated	1 Tbs	14	125	0	0	14	2.1	6.0	5.3	0
Soybean-cottonseed oil blend, partially hydrogenated	1 Tbs	14	125	0	0	14	2.5	4.1	6.7	0
Sunflower	1 Tbs	14	125	0	0	14	1.4	2.7	9.2	0
Salad dressings:										
Commercial:										
Blue cheese	1 Tbs	15	75	1	1	8	1.5	1.8	4.2	3
French:										
Regular	1 Tbs	16	85	tr	1	9	1.4	4.0	3.5	0
Low calorie	1 Tbs	16	25	tr	2	2	0.2	0.3	1.0	0
Italian:										
Regular	1 Tbs	15	80	tr	1	9	1.3	3.7	3.2	0
Low calorie	1 Tbs	15	5	tr	2	tr	tr	tr	tr	0
Mayonnaise:										
Regular	1 Tbs	14	100	tr	tr	11	1.7	3.2	5.8	8
Imitation	1 Tbs	15	35	tr	2	3	0.5	0.7	1.6	4
Mayonnaise type	1 Tbs	15	60	tr	4	5	0.7	1.4	2.7	4
Tartar	1 Tbs	14	75	tr	1	8	1.2	2.6	3.9	4

Fats and Oils continued

Foods	Approximate Measure Portion	Weight Grams	Calories Calories	Protein Grams	Carbohydrate Grams	Total Fat Grams	Fats Saturated Grams	Fats Mono-unsaturated Grams	Fats Poly-unsaturated Grams	Cholesterol Milligrams
Thousand island:										
Regular	1 Tbs	16	60	tr	2	6	1.0	1.3	3.2	4
Low calorie	1 Tbs	15	25	tr	2	2	0.2	0.4	0.9	2
Prepared from own recipe:										
Cooked type	1 Tbs	16	25	1	2	2	0.5	0.6	0.3	9
Vinegar & oil	1 Tbs	16	70	0	tr	8	1.5	2.4	3.9	0

Fish and Shellfish

Foods	Approximate Measure Portion	Weight Grams	Calories Calories	Protein Grams	Carbohydrate Grams	Total Fat Grams	Fats Saturated Grams	Fats Mono-unsaturated Grams	Fats Poly-unsaturated Grams	Cholesterol Milligrams
Clams:										
Raw, meat only	3 oz	85	65	11	2	1	0.3	0.3	0.3	43
Canned, drained	3 oz	85	85	13	2	2	0.5	0.5	0.4	54
Crabmeat, canned	1 cup	135	135	23	1	3	0.5	0.8	1.4	135
Fish sticks	1 stick	28	70	6	4	3	0.8	1.4	0.8	26
Flounder or Sole, baked with lemon juice:										
With butter	3 oz	85	120	16	tr	6	3.2	1.5	0.5	68
With margarine	3 oz	85	120	16	tr	6	1.2	2.3	1.9	59
Without added fat	3 oz	85	80	17	tr	1	0.3	0.2	0.4	55
Haddock, breaded, fried	3 oz	85	175	17	tr	9	2.4	3.9	2.4	75
Halibut, broiled, with butter & lemon juice	3 oz	85	140	20	tr	6	3.3	1.6	0.7	62
Herring, pickled	3 oz	85	190	17	0	13	4.3	4.6	3.1	85
Ocean perch, breaded, fried	1 fillet	85	185	16	7	11	2.6	4.6	2.8	66

Food	Amount									
Oysters:										
Raw, meat only	1 cup	240	160	20	8	4	1.4	0.5	1.4	120
Breaded, fried	1 oyster	45	90	5	5	5	1.4	2.1	1.4	35
Salmon:										
Canned (pink), solids & liquid	3 oz	85	120	17	0	5	0.9	1.5	2.1	34
Baked (red)	3 oz	85	140	21	0	5	1.2	2.4	1.4	60
Smoked	3 oz	85	150	18	0	8	2.6	3.9	0.7	51
Sardines, Atlantic, canned										
in oil, drained	3 oz	85	175	20	0	9	2.1	3.7	2.9	85
Scallops, breaded	6	90	195	15	10	10	2.5	4.1	2.5	70
Shrimp:										
Canned, drained	3 oz	85	100	21	1	1	0.2	0.2	0.4	128
French fried, 7 med.	3 oz	85	200	16	11	10	2.5	4.1	2.6	168
Trout, broiled, with butter										
and lemon juice	3 oz	85	175	21	tr	9	4.1	2.9	1.6	71
Tuna, canned, drained:										
Oil packed, chunk light	3 oz	85	165	24	0	7	1.4	1.9	3.1	55
Water packed, solid white	3 oz	85	135	30	0	1	0.3	0.2	0.3	48
Tuna salad	1 cup	205	375	33	19	19	3.3	4.9	9.2	80
Fruit and Fruit Juices										
Apples:										
Raw:										
Unpeeled, without core:										
2¾″ diam	1 apple	138	80	tr	21	tr	0.1	tr	0.1	0
3¼″ diam	1 apple	212	125	tr	32	1	0.1	tr	0.2	0
Peeled, sliced	1 cup	110	65	tr	16	tr	0.1	tr	0.1	0
Dried, sulfured	10 rings	64	155	1	42	tr	tr	tr	0.1	0
Apple juice	1 cup	248	115	tr	29	tr	tr	tr	0.1	0

Fruit and Fruit Juices continued

Foods	Approximate Measure (Portion)	Weight (Grams)	Calories (Calories)	Protein (Grams)	Carbohydrate (Grams)	Total Fat (Grams)	Fats Saturated (Grams)	Fats Mono-unsaturated (Grams)	Fats Poly-unsaturated (Grams)	Cholesterol (Milligrams)
Applesauce, canned:										
Sweetened	1 cup	255	195	tr	51	tr	0.1	tr	0.1	0
Unsweetened	1 cup	244	105	tr	28	tr	tr	tr	tr	0
Apricots:										
Raw	3	106	50	1	12	tr	tr	0.2	0.1	0
Canned (fruit & liquid):										
Heavy syrup pack	1 cup	258	215	1	55	tr	tr	0.1	tr	0
	3 halves	85	70	tr	18	tr	tr	tr	tr	0
Juice pack	1 cup	248	120	2	31	tr	tr	tr	tr	0
	3 halves	84	40	1	10	tr	tr	tr	tr	0
Dried:										
Uncooked	1 cup	130	310	5	80	1	tr	0.3	0.1	0
Cooked, unsweetened, fruit & liquid	1 cup	250	210	3	55	tr	tr	0.2	0.1	0
Apricot nectar	1 cup	251	140	1	36	tr	tr	0.1	tr	0
Avocados, raw:										
California, 2/lb	1 avocado	173	305	4	12	30	4.5	19.4	3.5	0
Florida, 1/lb	1 avocado	304	340	5	27	27	5.3	14.8	4.5	0
Bananas, 2 ½/lb	1 banana	114	105	1	27	1	0.2	tr	0.1	0
Sliced	1 cup	150	140	2	35	1	0.3	0.1	0.1	0
Blackberries, raw	1 cup	144	75	1	18	1	0.2	0.1	0.1	0
Blueberries:										
Raw	1 cup	145	80	1	20	1	tr	0.1	0.3	0
Frozen, sweetened	1 cup	230	185	1	50	tr	tr	tr	tr	0
Cantaloupe, 5" diam	½ melon	267	95	2	22	1	0.1	0.1	0.3	0

Food	Weight (g)	Food energy (cal.)	Protein (g)	Fat (g)				
Cherries:								
Sour, red, pitted, canned, water pack ....1 cup	244	90	2	tr	0.1	0.1	0.1	0
Sweet, raw 10	68	50	1	1	0.1	0.2	0.2	0
Cranberry juice cocktail,								
bottled, sweetened...............1 cup	253	145	tr	tr	tr	tr	0.1	0
Cranberry sauce, sweetened,								
canned, strained ....1 cup	277	420	1	tr	tr	0.1	0.2	0
Dates:								
Whole ....10 dates	83	230	2	tr	0.1	0.1	tr	0
Chopped...........................1 cup	178	490	4	1	0.3	0.2	tr	0
Figs, dried ....10 figs	187	475	6	2	0.4	0.5	1.0	0
Fruit cocktail, canned, fruit and liquid:								
Heavy syrup pack ....1 cup	255	185	1	tr	tr	tr	0.1	0
Juice pack ....1 cup	248	115	1	tr	tr	tr	tr	0
Grapefruit:								
Raw, 3¾″ diam ....½	120	40	1	tr	tr	tr	tr	0
Canned, with syrup..........1 cup	254	150	1	tr	tr	tr	0.1	0
Grapefruit juice:								
Fresh ....1 cup	247	95	1	tr	tr	tr	0.1	0
Canned:								
Unsweetened...................1 cup	247	95	1	tr	tr	tr	0.1	0
Sweetened ....1 cup	250	115	1	tr	tr	tr	0.1	0
Frozen concentrate, unsweetened:								
Undiluted.................6 oz can	207	300	4	1	0.1	0.1	0.2	0
Diluted with 3 parts water by volume.................1 cup	247	100	1	tr	tr	tr	0.1	0
Grapes, raw:								
Thompson Seedless ....10 grapes	50	35	tr	tr	0.1	tr	0.1	0

Fruit and Fruit Juices continued

Foods	Approximate Measure (Portion)	Weight (Grams)	Calories	Protein (Grams)	Carbohydrate (Grams)	Total Fat (Grams)	Saturated (Grams)	Mono-unsaturated (Grams)	Poly-unsaturated (Grams)	Cholesterol (Milligrams)
Tokay & Emperor, seeded types ....10 grapes		57	40	tr	10	tr	0.1	tr	0.1	0
Grape juice:										
Canned or bottled ....1 cup		253	155	1	38	tr	0.1	tr	0.1	0
Frozen concentrate, sweetened:										
Undiluted ....6 oz can		216	385	1	96	1	0.2	tr	0.2	0
Diluted with 3 parts water by volume............1 cup		250	125	tr	32	tr	0.1	tr	0.1	0
Honeydew, 6½″ diam............1/10 melon		129	45	1	12	tr	tr	tr	0.1	0
Kiwifruit, raw, 5/lb............1 kiwi		76	45	1	11	tr	tr	0.1	0.1	0
Lemons, 4/lb............1 lemon		58	15	1	5	tr	tr	tr	0.1	0
Lemon juice:										
Fresh ....1 cup		244	60	1	21	tr	tr	tr	tr	0
Canned or bottled, unsweetened ....1 cup		244	50	1	16	1	0.1	tr	0.2	0
............1 Tbs		15	5	tr	1	tr	tr	tr	tr	0
Frozen, single-strength, unsweetened ....6 oz can		244	55	1	16	1	0.1	tr	0.2	0
Lime juice:										
Fresh............1 cup		246	65	1	22	tr	tr	tr	0.1	0
Canned, unsweetened............1 cup		246	50	1	16	1	0.1	0.1	0.2	0
Mangos, 1½/lb............1 mango		207	135	1	35	1	0.1	0.2	0.1	0
Nectarines, 3/lb............1 nect.		136	65	1	16	1	0.1	0.2	0.3	0
Oranges:										
Whole, 2⅝″ diam............1 orange		131	60	1	15	tr	tr	tr	tr	0
sections ....1 cup		180	85	2	21	tr	r	tr	tr	0

Food	Measure									
Orange juice:										
Fresh	1 cup	248	110	2	26	tr	0.1	0.1	0.1	0
Canned, unsweetened	1 cup	249	105	1	25	tr	tr	0.1	0.1	0
Frozen concentrate:										
Undiluted	6 oz can	213	340	5	81	tr	0.1	0.1	0.1	0
Diluted, 3 parts water by volume	1 cup	249	110	2	27	tr	tr	tr	tr	0
Orange & grapefruit juice canned	1 cup	247	105	1	25	tr	tr	tr	tr	0
Papayas, raw, cubed	1 cup	140	65	1	17	tr	0.1	0.1	tr	0
Peaches:										
Raw, 2½″ diam	1 peach	87	35	1	10	tr	tr	tr	tr	0
Sliced	1 cup	170	75	1	19	tr	tr	0.1	0.1	0
Canned, fruit & liquid:										
Heavy syrup	1 cup	256	190	1	51	tr	tr	0.1	0.1	0
	½	81	60	tr	16	tr	tr	tr	tr	0
Juice pack	1 cup	248	110	2	29	tr	tr	tr	tr	0
	½	77	35	tr	9	tr	tr	tr	tr	0
Dried:										
Uncooked	1 cup	160	380	6	98	1	0.1	0.4	0.6	0
Cooked, unsweetened with liquid	1 cup	258	200	3	51	1	0.1	0.2	0.3	0
Frozen, sliced, sweetened	1 cup	250	235	2	60	tr	tr	0.1	0.2	0
Pears:										
Bartlett 2½″ diam	1 pear	166	100	1	25	1	tr	0.1	0.2	0
Bosc 2½″ diam	1 pear	141	85	1	21	1	tr	0.1	0.1	0
D'Anjou 3″ diam	1 pear	200	120	1	30	1	tr	0.2	0.2	0
Canned, fruit & liquid:										
Heavy syrup pack	1 cup	255	190	1	49	tr	tr	0.1	0.1	0
	½	79	60	tr	15	tr	tr	tr	tr	0

Fruit and Fruit Juices continued

Foods	Approximate Measure (Portion)	Weight Grams	Calories	Protein Grams	Carbohydrate Grams	Total Fat Grams	Fats Saturated Grams	Fats Mono-unsaturated Grams	Fats Poly-unsaturated Grams	Cholesterol Milligrams
Juice pack............	1 cup	248	125	1	32	tr	tr	tr	tr	0
	½	77	40	tr	10	tr	tr	tr	tr	0
Pineapple:										
Raw, diced............	1 cup	155	75	1	19	1	tr	0.1	0.2	0
Canned, fruit & liquid:										
Heavy syrup pack:										
Crushed, chunks, tibits........	1 cup	255	200	1	52	tr	tr	tr	0.1	0
Slices............	1 slice	58	45	tr	12	tr	tr	tr	tr	0
Juice pack:										
Crushed, chunks, tibits........	1 cup	250	150	1	39	tr	tr	tr	0.1	0
Slices............	1 slice	58	35	tr	9	tr	tr	tr	tr	0
Pineapple juice, unsweetened, canned............	1 cup	250	140	1	34	tr	tr	tr	tr	0
Plantains:										
Raw............	1	179	220	2	57	1	0.3	0.1	0.1	0
Cooked, sliced........	1 cup	154	180	1	48	tr	0.1	tr	0.1	0
Plums:										
Raw:										
2⅛″ diam............	1 plum	66	35	1	9	tr	tr	0.3	0.1	0
1½″ diam............	1 plum	28	15	tr	4	tr	tr	0.1	tr	0
Canned, purple, fruit and liquid:										
Heavy syrup pack	1 cup	258	230	1	60	tr	tr	0.2	0.1	0
	3 plums	133	120	tr	31	tr	tr	0.1	tr	0
Juice pack............	1 cup	252	145	1	38	tr	tr	tr	tr	0
	3 plums	95	55	tr	14	tr	tr	tr	tr	0

Food	Amount									
Prunes, dried:										
Uncooked	4 x-large or 5 large	49	115	1	31	tr	tr	0.2	0.1	0
Cooked, unsweetened, with liquid	1 cup	212	225	2	60	tr	tr	0.3	0.1	0
Prune juice, canned	1 cup	256	180	2	45	tr	tr	0.1	tr	0
Raisins, seedless:										
Not pressed down	1 cup	145	435	5	115	1	0.2	tr	0.2	0
Packet, ½ oz	1½ Tbs	14	40	tr	11	tr	tr	tr	tr	0
Raspberries:										
Raw	1 cup	123	60	1	14	1	tr	0.1	0.4	0
Frozen, sweetened	1 cup	250	255	2	65	tr	tr	tr	0.2	0
Rhubarb, cooked, sugar added	1 cup	240	280	1	75	tr	tr	tr	0.1	0
Strawberries:										
Raw, whole	1 cup	149	45	1	10	1	tr	0.1	0.3	0
Frozen, sweetened, sliced	1 cup	255	245	1	66	tr	tr	tr	0.2	0
Tangerines:										
Raw, 2⅜" diam	1 tangerine	84	35	1	9	tr	tr	tr	tr	0
Canned, light syrup, fruit & liquid	1 cup	252	155	1	41	tr	tr	tr	0.1	0
Tangerine juice, canned, sweetened	1 cup	249	125	1	30	tr	tr	tr	0.1	0
Watermelon, raw:										
4 x 8" wedge	1 piece	482	155	3	35	2	0.3	0.2	1.0	0
Diced	1 cup	160	50	1	11	1	0.1	0.1	0.3	0

Grain Products

Food	Amount									
Bagel, plain or water, enriched, 3½" diam	1 bagel	68	200	7	38	2	0.3	0.5	0.7	0

Grain Products continued

Foods	Approximate Measure	Weight	Calories	Protein	Carbohydrate	Total Fat	Fats Saturated	Fats Mono-unsaturated	Fats Poly-unsaturated	Cholesterol
	Portion	Grams	Calories	Grams	Grams	Grams	Grams	Grams	Grams	Milligrams
Barley, pearled, light uncooked ......1 cup	1 cup	200	700	16	158	2	0.3	0.2	0.9	0
Biscuits, baking powder 2″ diam (enriched flour, veg. short.):										
From home recipe .... 1 biscuit	1 biscuit	28	100	2	13	5	1.2	2.0	1.3	tr
From mix .... 1 biscuit	1 biscuit	28	95	2	14	3	0.8	1.4	0.9	tr
From refrig. dough .... 1 biscuit	1 biscuit	20	65	1	10	2	0.6	0.9	0.6	1
Breadcrumbs, enriched:										
Dry, grated ....1 cup	1 cup	100	390	13	73	5	1.5	1.6	1.0	5
Soft ....1 cup	1 cup	45	120	4	22	2	0.6	0.6	0.4	0
Breads:										
Boston Brown, canned, sliced ...... 1 slice	1 slice	45	95	2	21	1	0.3	0.1	0.1	3
Cracked-wheat .... 1 slice	1 slice	25	65	2	12	1	0.2	0.2	0.3	1
French 5 x 2½ x 1″ .... 1 slice	1 slice	35	100	3	18	1	0.3	0.4	0.5	0
Vienna 4¾ x 4 x ½″ .... 1 slice	1 slice	25	70	2	13	1	0.2	0.3	0.3	0
Italian 4½ x 3¼ x ¾″ .... 1 slice	1 slice	30	85	3	17	tr	tr	tr	0.1	0
Mixed grain, enriched:										
Slices, 18/loaf .... 1 slice	1 slice	25	65	2	12	1	0.2	0.2	0.4	0
Toasted .... 1 slice	1 slice	23	65	2	12	1	0.2	0.2	0.4	0
Oatmeal:										
Slices 18/loaf .... 1 slice	1 slice	25	65	2	12	1	0.2	0.4	0.5	0
Toasted .... 1 slice	1 slice	23	65	2	12	1	0.2	0.4	0.5	0
Pita 6½″ diam .... 1 pita	1 pita	60	165	6	33	1	0.1	0.1	0.4	0
Pumpernickel:										
Slice 5 x 4 x ⅜″ .... 1 slice	1 slice	32	80	3	16	1	0.2	0.3	0.5	0
Toasted .... 1 slice	1 slice	29	80	3	16	1	0.2	0.3	0.5	0

Food	Measure									
Raisin, enriched:										
Slice 18/loaf	1 slice	25	65	2	13	1	0.2	0.3	0.4	0
Toasted	1 slice	21	65	2	13	1	0.2	0.3	0.4	0
Rye, light:										
Slice 4¾ x 3¾ x 7/16	1 slice	25	65	2	12	1	0.2	0.3	0.3	0
Wheat bread, enriched:										
18 slices/loaf	1 slice	25	65	2	12	1	0.2	0.4	0.3	0
White bread, enriched:										
18 slices/loaf	1 slice	25	65	2	12	1	0.3	0.4	0.2	0
Cubes	1 cup	30	80	2	15	1	0.4	0.4	0.3	0
Whole Wheat:										
16 slices/loaf	1 slice	28	70	3	13	1	0.4	0.4	0.3	0
Bread stuffing, from mix:										
Dry type	1 cup	140	500	9	50	31	6.1	13.3	9.6	0
Moist type	1 cup	203	420	9	40	26	5.3	11.3	8.0	67
Breakfast cereals:										
Hot type:										
Corn (hominy) grits:										
Regular & enriched	1 cup	242	145	3	31	tr	tr	0.1	0.2	0
Instant, plain	1 pkt	137	80	2	18	tr	tr	tr	0.1	0
Cream of Wheat:										
Regular, quick, instant	1 cup	244	140	4	29	tr	0.1	tr	0.2	0
Mix'n Eat, plain	1 pkt.	142	100	3	21	tr	tr	tr	0.1	0
Malt-O-Meal	1 cup	240	120	4	26	tr	tr	tr	0.1	0
Oatmeal or rolled oats:										
Regular, quick, instant, nonfortified	1 cup	234	145	6	25	2	0.4	0.8	1.0	0
Instant, fortified:										
Plain	1 pkt	177	105	4	18	2	0.3	0.6	0.7	0
Flavored	1 pkt	164	160	5	31	2	0.3	0.7	0.8	0

Grain Products continued

Foods	Approximate Measure — Portion	Weight — Grams	Calories — Calories	Protein — Grams	Carbohydrate — Grams	Total Fat — Grams	Fats — Saturated — Grams	Fats — Mono-unsaturated — Grams	Fats — Poly-unsaturated — Grams	Cholesterol — Milligrams
Ready to eat:										
All-Bran	⅓ cup	28	70	4	21	1	0.1	0.1	0.3	0
Cap'n Crunch	¾ cup	28	120	1	23	3	1.7	0.3	0.4	0
Cheerios	1¼ cup	28	110	4	20	2	0.3	0.6	0.7	0
Corn Flakes:										
Kellogg's	1¼ cup	28	110	2	24	tr	tr	tr	tr	0
Toasties	1¼ cup	28	110	2	24	tr	tr	tr	tr	0
40% Bran Flakes:										
Kellogg's	¾ cup	28	90	4	22	1	0.1	0.1	0.3	0
Post	⅔ cup	28	90	3	22	tr	0.1	0.1	0.2	0
Froot Loops	1 cup	28	110	2	25	1	0.2	0.1	0.1	0
Golden Grahams	¾ cup	28	110	2	24	1	0.7	0.1	0.2	tr
Grape-Nuts	¼ cup	28	100	3	23	tr	tr	tr	0.1	0
Honey Nut Cheerios	¾ cup	28	105	3	23	1	0.1	0.3	0.3	0
Lucky Charms	1 cup	28	110	3	23	1	0.2	0.4	0.4	0
Nature Valley Granola	⅓ cup	28	125	3	19	5	3.3	0.7	0.7	0
100% Natural Cereal	¼ cup	28	135	3	18	6	4.1	1.2	0.5	tr
Product 19	¾ cup	28	110	3	24	tr	tr	tr	0.1	0
Raisin Bran:										
Kellogg's	¾ cup	28	90	3	21	1	0.1	0.1	0.3	0
Post	½ cup	28	85	3	21	1	0.1	0.1	0.3	0
Rice Krispies	1 cup	28	110	2	25	tr	tr	tr	0.1	0
Shredded Wheat	⅔ cup	28	100	3	23	1	0.1	0.1	0.3	0
Special K	1⅓ cup	28	110	6	21	tr	tr	tr	tr	tr

Food	Measure									
Super Sugar Crisp	⅞ cup	28	105	2	26	tr	tr	tr	0.1	0
Sugar Frosted Flakes:										
Kellogg's	¾ cup	28	110	1	26	tr	tr	tr	tr	0
Sugar Smacks	¾ cup	28	105	2	25	1	0.1	0.1	0.2	0
Total	1 cup	28	100	3	22	1	0.1	0.1	0.3	0
Trix	1 cup	28	110	2	25	tr	0.2	0.1	0.1	0
Wheaties	1 cup	28	100	3	23	tr	0.1	tr	0.2	0
Buckwheat flour, light, sifted	1 cup	98	340	6	78	1	0.2	0.4	0.4	0
Bulgur, uncooked	1 cup	170	600	19	129	3	1.2	0.3	1.2	0
Cakes:										
Cakes prepared from mixes:										
Angelfood, 9¾" diam.										
¹⁄₁₂ of cake	1 slice	53	125	3	29	tr	tr	tr	0.1	0
Coffeecake, crumb 7¾ x 5⅝ × 1¼:										
⅙ of cake	1 slice	72	230	5	38	7	2.0	2.8	1.6	47
Devil's food 9" diam., chocolate										
icing: ¹⁄₁₆ of cake	1 slice	69	235	3	40	8	3.5	3.2	1.2	37
Cupcake, 2½" diam.	1 cupcake	35	120	2	20	4	1.8	1.6	0.6	19
Gingerbread, 8" sq.:										
⅑ of cake	1 piece	63	175	2	32	4	1.1	1.8	1.2	1
Yellow 9" diam., chocolate										
icing: ¹⁄₁₆ of cake	1 piece	69	235	3	40	8	3.0	3.0	1.4	36
Cakes prepared from home recipe:										
Carrot, 10" diam with cream cheese icing:										
¹⁄₁₆ cake	1 piece	96	385	4	48	21	4.1	8.4	6.7	74
Fruitcake, dark, tube cake:										
¹⁄₃₂ of cake	1 piece	43	165	2	25	7	1.5	3.6	1.6	20

Grain Products continued

Foods	Approximate Measure (Portion)	Weight (Grams)	Calories	Protein (Grams)	Carbohydrate (Grams)	Total Fat (Grams)	Saturated (Grams)	Mono-unsaturated (Grams)	Poly-unsaturated (Grams)	Cholesterol (Milligrams)
Plain sheet cake, 9" sq.:										
Without icing:										
⅑ of cake................	1 piece	86	315	4	48	12	3.3	5.0	2.8	61
With uncooked white icing:										
⅑ of cake:	1 piece	121	445	4	77	14	4.6	5.6	2.9	70
Pound, 8½ x 3½ x 3¼":										
1/17 of loaf..............	1 slice	30	120	2	15	5	1.2	2.4	1.6	32
Cakes, commercial:										
Pound, 8½ x 3½ x 3":										
1/17 of loaf.............	1 slice	29	110	2	15	5	3.0	1.7	0.2	64
Snack cakes:										
Devil's food with cream filling, 2/pack............	1 cake	28	105	1	17	4	1.7	1.5	0.6	15
Sponge with cream filling 2/pack	1 cake	42	155	1	27	5	2.3	2.1	0.5	7
White, 8 or 9" diam. with white icing: 1/16 of cake........	1 piece	71	260	3	42	9	2.1	3.8	2.6	3
Yellow, 8 or 9" diam. with chocolate icing; 1/16 of cake	1 piece	69	245	2	39	11	5.7	3.7	0.6	38
Cheesecake, 9" diam.: 1/12 of cake...............	1 piece	92	280	5	26	18	9.9	5.4	1.2	170

Food	Amount									
Cookies:										
Brownies with nuts:										
Commercial with icing,										
1½ x 1¾ x ⅞"	1 brownie	25	100	1	16	4	1.6	2.0	0.6	14
Home recipe, 1¾ x 1¾ x ⅞"	1 brownie	20	95	1	11	6	1.4	2.8	1.2	18
Chocolate chip:										
Commercial, 2¼" diam.										
⅜" thick	4 cookies	42	180	2	28	9	2.9	3.1	2.6	5
Home recipe, 2⅓" diam	4 cookies	40	185	2	26	11	3.9	4.3	2.0	18
From refrig. dough,										
2¼" diam	4 cookies	48	225	2	32	11	4.0	4.4	2.0	22
Fig bars, square,1⅝ x 1⅝ x ⅜"	4 cookies	56	210	2	42	4	1.0	1.5	1.0	27
Oatmeal with raisins,										
2⅝" diam	4 cookies	52	245	3	36	10	2.5	4.5	2.8	2
Peanut butter cookie,										
home recipe, 2⅝" diam	4 cookies	48	245	4	28	14	4.0	5.8	2.8	22
Sandwich type, choc. or vanilla,										
1¾" diam., ⅜" thick	4 cookies	40	195	2	29	8	2.0	3.6	2.2	0
Shortbread:										
Commercial	4 sm. cookies	32	155	2	20	8	2.9	3.0	1.1	27
Home recipe	2 lg. cookies	28	145	2	17	8	1.3	2.7	3.4	0
Sugar cookie, from refrig. dough										
2½" diam., ¼" thick	4 cookies	48	235	2	31	12	2.3	5.0	3.6	29
Vanilla wafers,										
1¾" diam., ¼" thick	10 cookies	40	185	2	29	7	1.8	3.0	1.8	25
Corn chips	1 oz pack.	28	155	2	16	9	1.4	2.4	3.7	0
Cornmeal:										
Whole-ground, unbolted,										
dry form	1 cup	122	435	11	90	5	0.5	1.1	2.5	0

Grain Products continued

Foods	Approximate Measure Portion	Weight Grams	Calories	Protein Grams	Carbohydrate Grams	Total Fat Grams	Fats Saturated Grams	Mono-unsaturated Grams	Poly-unsaturated Grams	Cholesterol Milligrams
Bolted, dry form............1 cup		122	440	11	91	4	0.5	0.9	2.2	0
Degermed, enriched:										
Dry form............1 cup		138	500	11	108	2	0.2	0.4	0.9	0
Cooked............1 cup		240	120	3	26	tr	tr	0.1	0.2	0
Crackers:										
Cheese:										
Plain, 1" sq............10 crackers		10	50	1	6	3	0.9	1.2	0.3	6
Sandwich type, peanut butter............ 1 sandwich		8	40	1	5	2	0.4	0.8	0.3	1
Graham, plain, 2½" sq ....2 crackers		14	60	1	11	1	0.4	0.6	0.4	0
Melba toast, plain............ 1 piece		5	20	1	4	tr	0.1	0.1	0.1	0
Rye wafers, whole-grain, 1⅞ x 3½" ....2 wafers		14	55	1	10	1	0.3	0.4	0.3	0
Saltines ....4 crackers		12	50	1	9	1	0.5	0.4	0.2	4
Snack type, standard cracker.... 1 round		3	15	tr	2	1	0.2	0.4	0.1	0
Wheat, thin ....4 crackers		8	35	1	5	1	0.5	0.5	0.4	0
Whole-wheat wafers ....2 crackers		8	35	1	5	2	0.5	0.6	0.4	0
Croissants 4½ x 4 x 1¾" ....1 croissant		57	235	5	27	12	3.5	6.7	1.4	13
Danish pastry:										
Plain without fruit or nuts:										
Round piece 4¼" diam., 1" high............ 1 pastry		57	220	4	26	12	3.6	4.8	2.6	49
Ounce............1 oz		28	110	2	13	6	1.8	2.4	1.3	24
Fruit, round piece............ 1 pastry		65	235	4	28	13	3.9	5.2	2.9	56

Food	Measure	(g)	cal	prot	carb	fat				
Doughnuts:										
Cake type, plain, 3¼" diam., 1" high	1 doughnut	50	210	3	24	12	2.8	5.0	3.0	20
Yeast type, glazed, 3¾" diam., 1" high	1 doughnut	60	235	4	26	13	5.2	5.5	0.9	21
English muffin, plain	1 muffin	57	140	5	27	1	0.3	0.2	0.3	0
French toast, home recipe	1 slice	65	155	6	17	7	1.6	2.0	1.6	112
Macaroni, enriched, cooked (shells, elbows)										
Firm stage	1 cup	130	190	7	39	1	0.1	0.1	0.3	0
Tender stage:										
Cold	1 cup	105	115	4	24	tr	0.1	0.1	0.2	0
Hot	1 cup	140	155	5	32	1	0.1	0.1	0.2	0
Muffins made with enriched flour, 2½" diam										
Home recipe										
Blueberry	1 muffin	45	135	3	20	5	1.5	2.1	1.2	19
Bran	1 muffin	45	125	3	19	6	1.4	1.6	2.3	24
Corn (enriched degermed cornmeal & flour)	1 muffin	45	145	3	21	5	1.5	2.2	1.4	23
From mix (egg & water added):										
Blueberry	1 muffin	45	140	3	22	5	1.4	2.0	1.2	45
Bran	1 muffin	45	140	3	24	4	1.3	1.6	1.0	28
Corn	1 muffin	45	145	3	22	6	1.7	2.3	1.4	42
Noodles (egg) enriched, cooked	1 cup	160	200	7	37	2	0.5	0.6	0.6	50
Noodles, chow mein, canned	1 cup	45	220	6	26	11	2.1	7.3	0.4	5
Pancakes, 4" diam.:										
Buckwheat, from mix, egg & milk added	1 pancake	27	55	2	6	2	0.9	0.9	0.5	20

Grain Products continued

Foods	Approximate Measure	Weight	Calories	Protein	Carbohydrate	Total Fat	Fats Saturated	Fats Mono-unsaturated	Fats Poly-unsaturated	Cholesterol
	Portion	Grams	Calories	Grams	Grams	Grams	Grams	Grams	Grams	Milligrams
Plain:										
Home recipe	1 pancake	27	60	2	9	2	0.5	0.8	0.5	16
Mix, egg, milk & oil added............	1 pancake	27	60	2	8	2	0.5	0.9	0.5	16
Piecrust, made with enriched flour, & veg. short., baked:										
Home recipe, 9" diam...........	1 pie shell	180	900	11	79	60	14.8	25.9	15.7	0
From mix, 9" diam	piecrust for 2 crust pie	320	1,485	20	141	93	22.7	41.0	25.0	0
Pies, crust made with enriched flour & veg. short., 9" diam.:										
Apple, ⅙ pie	1 piece	158	405	3	60	18	4.6	7.4	4.4	0
Blueberry, ⅙ pie	1 piece	158	380	4	55	17	4.3	7.4	4.6	0
Cherry, ⅙ pie	1 piece	158	410	4	61	18	4.7	7.7	4.6	0
Creme, ⅙ pie	1 piece	152	455	3	59	23	15.0	4.0	1.1	8
Custard, ⅙ pie	1 piece	152	330	9	36	17	5.6	6.7	3.2	169
Lemon meringue, ⅙ pie ...	1 piece	140	355	5	53	14	4.3	5.7	2.9	143
Peach, ⅙ pie...........	1 piece	158	405	4	60	17	4.1	7.3	4.4	0
Pecan, ⅙ pie...........	1 piece	138	575	7	71	32	4.7	17.0	7.9	95
Pumpkin, ⅙ pie..........	1 piece	152	320	6	37	17	6.4	6.7	3.0	109
Pies, fried:										
Apple............	1 pie	85	255	2	31	14	5.8	6.6	0.6	14
Cherry............	1 pie	85	250	2	32	14	5.8	6.7	0.6	13
Popcorn, popped:										
Air-popped, unsalted	1 cup	8	30	1	6	tr	tr	0.1	0.2	0

Food	Amount									
Popped in veg. oil, salted	1 cup	11	55	1	6	3	0.5	1.4	1.2	0
Sugar syrup coated	1 cup	35	135	2	30	1	0.1	0.3	0.6	0
Pretzels:										
Stick, 2¼" long	10 sticks	3	10	tr	2	tr	tr	tr	tr	0
Twisted, dutch, 2¾ x 2⅝"	1 pretzel	16	65	2	13	1	0.1	0.2	0.2	0
Twisted, thin, 3¼ x 2¼ x ¼"	10 pretzels	60	240	6	48	2	0.4	0.8	0.6	0
Rice:										
Brown, cooked, hot	1 cup	195	230	5	50	1	0.3	0.3	0.4	0
White:										
Commercial varieties, all types:										
Raw	1 cup	185	670	12	149	1	0.2	0.2	0.3	0
Cooked, served hot	1 cup	205	225	4	50	tr	0.1	0.1	0.1	0
Instant, ready-to-serve, hot	1 cup	165	180	4	40	0	0.1	0.1	0.1	0
Parboiled:										
Raw	1 cup	185	685	14	150	1	0.1	0.1	0.2	0
Cooked, served hot	1 cup	175	185	4	41	tr	tr	tr	0.1	0
Rolls, enriched:										
Commercial:										
Dinner, 2½" diam., 2" high	1 roll	28	85	2	14	2	0.5	0.8	0.6	tr
Frankfurter & hamburger (8/pk)	1 roll	40	115	3	20	2	0.5	0.8	0.6	tr
Hard, 3⅜" diam., 2" high	1 roll	50	155	5	30	2	0.4	0.5	0.6	tr
Hoagie, 11½ x 3 x 2½"	1 roll	135	400	11	72	8	1.8	3.0	2.2	tr
From home recipe:										
Dinner 2½ diam., 2" high	1 roll	35	120	3	20	3	0.8	1.2	0.9	12
Spaghetti, enriched, cooked:										
Firm stage, "al dente," served hot	1 cup	130	190	7	39	1	0.1	0.1	0.3	0
Tender stage, served hot	1 cup	140	155	5	32	1	0.1	0.1	0.2	0
Toaster pastries	1 pastry	54	210	2	38	6	1.7	3.6	0.4	0

Grain Products continued

Foods	Approximate Measure — Portion	Weight — Grams	Calories	Protein — Grams	Carbohydrate — Grams	Total Fat — Grams	Fats — Saturated — Grams	Fats — Mono-unsaturated — Grams	Fats — Poly-unsaturated — Grams	Cholesterol — Milligrams
Tortilla, corn	1 tortilla	30	65	2	13	1	0.1	0.3	0.6	0
Waffles, made with enriched flour, 7" diam.:										
Home recipe	1 waffle	75	245	7	26	13	4.0	4.9	2.6	102
From mix, egg & milk added.....	1 waffle	75	205	7	27	8	2.7	2.9	1.5	59
Wheat flours:										
All-purpose, enriched:										
Sifted, spooned............	1 cup	115	420	12	88	1	0.2	0.1	0.5	0
Unsifted, spooned	1 cup	125	455	13	95	1	0.2	0.1	0.5	0
Cake or pastry flour.........	1 cup	96	350	7	76	1	0.1	0.1	0.3	0
Self-rising, enriched, unsifted, spooned.........	1 cup	125	440	12	93	1	0.2	0.1	0.5	0
Whole wheat, from hard wheats, stirred	1 cup	120	400	16	85	2	0.3	0.3	1.1	0

Legumes, Nuts and Seeds

Foods	Approximate Measure — Portion	Weight — Grams	Calories	Protein — Grams	Carbohydrate — Grams	Total Fat — Grams	Fats — Saturated — Grams	Fats — Mono-unsaturated — Grams	Fats — Poly-unsaturated — Grams	Cholesterol — Milligrams
Almonds, shelled:										
Slivered, packed............	1 cup	135	795	27	28	70	6.7	45.8	14.8	0
Whole....................	1 oz	28	167	6	6	15	1.4	9.6	3.1	0
Beans, dry:										
Cooked, drained:										
Black	1 cup	171	225	15	41	1	0.1	0.1	0.5	0
Great Northern	1 cup	180	210	14	38	1	0.1	0.1	0.6	0
Lima....................	1 cup	190	260	16	49	1	0.2	0.1	0.5	0

Food	Measure	Grams	Cal							
Pea (navy)	1 cup	190	225	15	40	1	0.1	0.1	0.7	0
Pinto	1 cup	180	265	15	49	1	0.1	0.1	0.5	0
Canned, solids & liquid:										
White with:										
Frankfurters	1 cup	255	365	19	32	18	7.4	8.8	0.7	30
Pork & tomato sauce	1 cup	255	310	16	48	7	2.4	2.7	0.7	10
Pork & sweet sauce	1 cup	255	385	16	54	12	4.3	4.9	1.2	10
Red kidney	1 cup	255	230	15	42	1	0.1	0.1	0.6	0
Blacked-eyed peas, dry, cooked (with residual cooking liquid)	1 cup	250	190	13	35	1	0.2	tr	0.3	0
Brazil nuts, shelled	1 oz	28	185	4	4	19	4.6	6.5	6.8	0
Carob flour	1 cup	140	255	6	126	tr	tr	0.1	0.1	0
Cashews nuts, salted:										
Dry roasted	1 cup	137	785	21	45	63	12.5	37.4	10.7	0
	1 oz	28	165	4	9	13	2.6	7.7	2.2	0
Roasted in oil	1 cup	130	750	21	37	63	12.4	36.9	10.6	0
	1 oz	28	165	5	8	14	2.7	8.1	2.3	0
Chestnuts, European, roasted, shelled	1 cup	143	350	5	76	3	0.6	1.1	1.2	0
Chickpeas, cooked, drained	1 cup	163	270	15	45	4	0.4	0.9	1.9	0
Coconut:										
Raw:										
Piece, 2 x 2 x ½″	1 piece	45	160	1	7	15	13.4	0.6	0.2	0
Shredded or grated	1 cup	80	285	3	12	27	23.8	1.1	0.3	0
Dried, sweetened, shredded	1 cup	93	470	3	44	33	29.3	1.4	0.4	0
Filberts (hazelnuts), chopped	1 cup	115	725	15	18	72	5.3	56.5	6.9	0
	1 oz	28	180	4	4	18	1.3	13.9	1.7	0
Lentils, dry cooked	1 cup	200	215	16	38	1	0.1	0.2	0.5	0
Macadamia nuts, roasted in oil, salted	1 cup	134	960	10	17	103	15.4	80.9	1.8	0
	1 oz	28	205	2	4	22	3.2	17.1	0.4	0

Legumes, Nuts and Seeds continued

Foods	Approximate Measure	Weight	Calories	Protein	Carbohydrate	Total Fat	Fats			Cholesterol
							Saturated	Mono-unsaturated	Poly-unsaturated	
	Portion	Grams	Calories	Grams	Grams	Grams	Grams	Grams	Grams	Milligrams
Mixed nuts, with peanuts, salted:										
Dry roasted ....1 oz		28	170	5	7	15	2.0	8.9	3.1	0
Roasted in oil...........1 oz		28	175	5	6	16	2.5	9.0	3.8	0
Peanuts, roasted in oil, salted........1 cup		145	840	39	27	71	9.9	35.5	22.6	0
1 oz		28	165	8	5	14	1.9	6.9	4.4	0
Peanut butter............1 Tbs		16	95	5	3	8	1.4	4.0	2.5	0
Peas, split, dry, cooked............1 cup		200	230	16	42	1	0.1	0.1	0.3	0
Pecans, halves............1 cup		108	720	8	20	73	5.9	45.5	18.1	0
...........1 oz		28	190	2	5	19	1.5	12.0	4.7	0
Pine nuts (pinyons), shelled ....1 oz		28	160	3	5	17	2.7	6.5	7.3	0
Pistachio nuts, dried, shelled ....1 oz		28	165	6	7	14	1.7	9.3	2.1	0
Pumpkin & squash kernels, dry, hulled...........1 oz		28	155	7	5	13	2.5	4.0	5.9	0
Refried beans, canned...........1 cup		290	295	18	51	3	0.4	0.6	1.4	0
Sesame seeds, dry, hulled ....1 Tbs		8	45	2	1	4	0.6	1.7	1.9	0
Soybeans, dry, cooked, drained ....1 cup		180	235	20	19	10	1.3	1.9	5.3	0
Soybean products:										
Miso...........1 cup		276	470	29	65	13	1.8	2.6	7.3	0
Tofu, piece 2½ x 2¾ x 1" ....1 piece		120	85	9	3	5	0.7	1.0	2.9	0
Sunflower seeds, dry, hulled...........1 oz		28	160	6	5	14	1.5	2.7	9.3	0
Tahini ....1 Tbs		15	90	3	3	8	1.1	3.0	3.5	0
Walnuts:										
Black, chopped ....1 cup		125	760	30	15	71	4.5	15.9	46.9	0
...........1 oz		28	170	7	3	16	1.0	3.6	10.6	0

Food	Measure									
English or Persian, chips	1 cup	120	770	17	22	74	6.7	17.0	47.0	0
	1 oz	28	180	4	5	18	1.6	4.0	11.1	0

Meats and Meat Products

Beef, cooked:

Cuts braised, simmered, or pot roasted:

Relatively fat such as chuck blade:

Food	Measure									
Lean & fat, piece	3 oz	85	325	22	0	26	10.8	11.7	0.9	87
Lean only	2.2 oz	62	170	19	0	9	3.9	4.2	0.3	66

Relatively lean, such as bottom round:

Food	Measure									
Lean & fat	3 oz	85	220	25	0	13	4.8	5.7	0.5	81
Lean only	2.8 oz	78	175	25	0	8	2.7	3.4	0.3	75

Ground beef, broiled patty:

Food	Measure									
Lean	3 oz	85	230	21	0	16	6.2	6.9	0.6	74
Regular	3 oz	85	245	20	0	18	6.9	7.7	0.7	76
Heart, lean, braised	3 oz	85	150	24	0	5	1.2	0.8	1.6	164
Liver, fried	3 oz	85	185	23	7	7	2.5	3.6	1.3	410

Roast, oven cooked, no liquid added:

Relatively fat, such as rib:

Food	Measure									
Lean & fat	3 oz	85	315	19	0	26	10.8	11.4	0.9	72
Lean only	2.2 oz	61	150	17	0	9	3.6	3.7	0.3	49

Relatively lean, such as eye of round:

Food	Measure									
Lean & fat	3 oz	85	205	23	0	12	4.9	5.4	0.5	62
Lean only	2.6 oz	75	135	22	0	5	1.9	2.1	0.2	52

Steak:

Sirloin broiled:

Food	Measure									
Lean & fat	3 oz	85	240	23	0	15	6.4	6.9	0.6	77
Lean only	2.5 oz	72	150	22	0	6	2.6	2.8	0.3	64

Foods	Approximate Measure	Weight	Calories	Protein	Carbohydrate	Total Fat	Fats Saturated	Fats Mono-unsaturated	Fats Poly-unsaturated	Cholesterol
	Portion	Grams	Calories	Grams	Grams	Grams	Grams	Grams	Grams	Milligrams
Meats and Meat Products continued										
Beef, canned, corned	3 oz	85	185	22	0	10	4.2	4.9	0.4	80
Beef, dried, chipped	2.5 oz	72	145	24	0	4	1.8	2.0	0.2	46
Lamb, cooked:										
Chops:										
Arm, braised:										
Lean & fat	2.2 oz	63	220	20	0	15	6.9	6.0	0.9	77
Lean only	1.7 oz	48	135	17	0	7	2.9	2.6	0.4	59
Loin, broiled:										
Lean & fat	2.8 oz	80	235	22	0	16	7.3	6.4	1.0	78
Lean only	2.3 oz	64	140	19	0	6	2.6	2.4	0.4	60
Leg, roasted:										
Lean & fat	3 oz	85	205	22	0	13	5.6	4.9	0.8	78
Lean only	2.6 oz	73	140	20	0	6	2.4	2.2	0.4	65
Rib roasted:										
Lean & fat	3 oz	85	315	18	0	26	12.1	10.1	1.5	77
Lean only	2 oz	57	130	15	0	7	3.2	3.0	0.5	50
Pork, cured, cooked:										
Bacon:										
Regular	3 med slices	19	110	6	tr	9	3.3	4.5	1.1	16
Canadian-style	2 slices	46	85	11	1	4	1.3	1.9	0.4	27
Ham, light cure, roasted:										
Lean & fat	3 oz	85	205	18	0	14	5.1	6.7	1.5	53
Lean only	2.4 oz	68	105	17	0	4	1.3	1.7	0.4	37
Ham, canned, roasted	3 oz	85	140	18	tr	7	2.4	3.5	0.8	35

Food	Measure									
Luncheon meat:										
Canned, 3 x 2 x ½	2 slices	42	140	5	1	13	4.5	6.0	1.5	26
Chopped ham, 8 slices/6 oz. pack	2 slices	42	95	7	0	7	2.4	3.4	0.9	21
Cooked ham, 8 slices/6 oz pack:										
Regular	2 slices	57	105	10	2	6	1.9	2.8	0.7	32
Extra lean	2 slices	57	75	11	1	3	0.9	1.3	0.3	27
Pork, fresh, cooked:										
Chop, loin:										
Broiled:										
Lean & fat	3.1 oz	87	275	24	0	19	7.0	8.8	2.2	84
Lean only	2.5 oz	72	165	23	0	8	2.6	3.4	0.9	71
Pan fried:										
Lean & fat	3.1 oz	89	335	21	0	27	9.8	12.5	3.1	92
Lean only	2.4 oz	67	180	19	0	11	3.7	4.8	1.3	72
Ham (leg) roasted:										
Lean & fat	3 oz	85	250	21	0	18	6.4	8.1	2.0	79
Lean only	2.5 oz	72	160	20	0	8	2.7	3.6	1.0	68
Rib, roasted:										
Lean & fat	3 oz	85	270	21	0	20	7.2	9.2	2.3	69
Lean only	2.5 oz	71	175	20	0	10	3.4	4.4	1.2	56
Shoulder cut, braised:										
Lean & fat	3 oz	85	295	23	0	22	7.9	10.0	2.4	93
Lean only	2.4 oz	67	165	22	0	8	2.8	3.7	1.0	76
Sausages:										
Bologna, 8 slices/8 oz. pack	2 slices	57	180	7	2	16	6.1	7.6	1.4	31
Braunschweiger, 6 slices/6 oz. pack	2 slices	57	205	8	2	18	6.2	8.5	2.1	89
Brown & serve, 10–11/8 oz. pack	1 link	13	50	2	tr	5	1.7	2.2	0.5	9
Frankfurter, 10/lb	1 frank	45	145	5	1	13	4.8	6.2	1.2	23

Meat and Meat Products continued

Foods	Approximate Measure Portion	Weight Grams	Calories Calories	Protein Grams	Carbohydrate Grams	Total Fat Grams	Saturated Grams	Fats Mono- unsaturated Grams	Poly- unsaturated Grams	Cholesterol Milligrams
Pork link, 16/lb .... 1 link		13	50	3	tr	4	1.4	1.8	0.5	11
Salami:										
Cooked type, 8 slices/										
8 oz. pack.................. 2 slices		57	145	8	1	11	4.6	5.2	1.2	37
Dry type, slice, 12/4 oz pack .... 2 slices		20	85	5	1	7	2.4	3.4	0.6	16
Sandwich spread (pork, beef) ......1 Tbs		15	35	1	2	3	0.9	1.1	0.4	6
Vienna sausage, 7/4 oz ....1 sausage		16	45	2	tr	4	1.5	2.0	0.3	8
Veal, medium fat, cooked:										
Cutlet, broiled ....3 oz		85	185	23	0	9	4.1	4.1	0.6	109
Rib, roasted ....3 oz		85	230	23	0	14	6.0	6.0	1.0	109

Mixed Dishes and Fast Food

Foods	Approximate Measure Portion	Weight Grams	Calories Calories	Protein Grams	Carbohydrate Grams	Total Fat Grams	Saturated Grams	Fats Mono- unsaturated Grams	Poly- unsaturated Grams	Cholesterol Milligrams
Mixed dishes:										
Beef and vegetable stew,										
from home recipe ....1 cup		245	220	16	15	11	4.4	4.5	0.5	71
Beef potpie, home recipe,										
⅓ of 9" diam. pie............. 1 piece		210	515	21	39	30	7.9	12.9	7.4	42
Chicken a la king, home recipe.....1 cup		245	470	27	12	34	12.9	13.4	6.2	221
Chicken & Noodles, cooked										
from home recipe..............1 cup		240	365	22	26	18	5.1	7.1	3.9	103
Chicken chow mein:										
Canned ....1 cup		250	95	7	18	tr	0.1	0.1	0.8	8
Home recipe ....1 cup		250	255	31	10	10	4.1	4.9	3.5	75
Chicken potpie, home recipe										
⅓ of 9" pie.................. 1 piece		232	545	23	42	31	10.3	15.5	6.6	56

Food	Measure								
Chili con carne with beans, canned	1 cup	255	340	19	31	16	5.8	7.2	1.0	28
Chop suey with beef & pork, home recipe	1 cup	250	300	26	13	17	4.3	7.4	4.2	68
Macaroni & cheese:										
Canned	1 cup	240	230	9	26	10	4.7	2.9	1.3	24
Home recipe	1 cup	200	430	17	40	22	9.8	7.4	3.6	44
Quiche Lorraine, ⅛ of 8" quiche	1 slice	176	600	13	29	48	23.2	17.8	4.1	285
Spaghetti in tomato sauce with cheese:										
Canned	1 cup	250	190	6	39	2	0.4	0.4	0.5	3
Home recipe	1 cup	250	260	9	37	9	3.0	3.6	1.2	8
Spaghetti with meatballs and tomato sauce:										
Canned	1 cup	250	260	12	29	10	2.4	3.9	3.1	23
Home recipe	1 cup	248	330	19	39	12	3.9	4.4	2.2	89
Fast food entrees:										
Cheeseburger:										
Regular	1 sandwich	112	300	15	28	15	7.3	5.6	1.0	44
4 oz. patty	1 sandwich	194	525	30	40	31	15.1	12.2	1.4	104
Chicken, fried. See Poultry & poultry products.										
Enchilada	1 enchilada	230	235	20	24	16	7.7	6.7	0.6	19
English muffin, egg, & bacon	1 sandwich	138	360	18	31	18	8.0	8.0	0.7	213
Fish sandwich:										
Regular, with cheese	1 sandwich	140	420	16	39	23	6.3	6.9	7.7	56
Large, no cheese	1 sandwich	170	470	18	41	27	6.3	8.7	9.5	91
Hamburger:										
Regular	1 sandwich	98	245	12	28	11	4.4	5.3	0.5	32
4 oz. patty	1 sandwich	174	445	25	38	21	7.1	11.7	0.6	71

Foods	Approximate Measure Portion	Weight Grams	Calories Calories	Protein Grams	Carbohydrate Grams	Total Fat Grams	Fats Saturated Grams	Mono-unsaturated Grams	Poly-unsaturated Grams	Cholesterol Milligrams

Mixed Dishes and Fast Food

Foods	Portion	Weight	Calories	Protein	Carbohydrate	Total Fat	Saturated	Mono-unsaturated	Poly-unsaturated	Cholesterol
Pizza, cheese, ⅛ of 15" diam. pizza	1 slice	120	290	15	39	9	4.1	2.6	1.3	56
Roast beef sandwich	1 sandwich	150	345	22	34	13	3.5	6.9	1.8	55
Taco	1 taco	81	195	9	15	11	4.1	5.5	0.8	21

Poultry and Poultry Products

Chicken:
Fried, flesh, with skin:
Batter dipped:

Foods	Portion	Weight	Calories	Protein	Carbohydrate	Total Fat	Saturated	Mono-unsaturated	Poly-unsaturated	Cholesterol
½ breast, 5.6 oz with bones	4.9 oz	140	365	35	13	18	4.9	7.6	4.3	119
Drumstick, 3.4 oz with bones	2.5 oz	72	195	16	6	11	3.0	4.6	2.7	62

Flour coated:

Foods	Portion	Weight	Calories	Protein	Carbohydrate	Total Fat	Saturated	Mono-unsaturated	Poly-unsaturated	Cholesterol
½ breast, 4.2 oz with bones	3.5 oz	98	220	31	2	9	2.4	3.4	1.9	87
Drumstick, 2.6 oz with bones	1.7 oz	49	120	13	1	7	1.8	2.7	1.6	44

Roasted, flesh only

Foods	Portion	Weight	Calories	Protein	Carbohydrate	Total Fat	Saturated	Mono-unsaturated	Poly-unsaturated	Cholesterol
½ breast, 4.2 oz with bones & skin	3.0 oz	86	140	27	0	3	0.9	1.1	0.7	73
Drumstick, 2.9 oz with bones & skin	1.6 oz	44	75	12	0	2	0.7	0.8	0.6	41
Stewed, flesh only, chopped or diced	1 cup	140	250	38	0	9	2.6	3.3	2.2	116
Chicken liver, cooked	1 liver	20	30	5	tr	1	0.4	0.3	0.2	126

Food (approximate measure)									
Duck, roasted, flesh only .... ½ duck	221	445	52	0	25	9.2	8.2	3.2	197
Turkey, roasted, flesh only:									
Dark meat, piece, 2½ x 1⅝ x ¼" ...... 4 pieces	85	160	24	0	6	2.1	1.4	1.8	72
Light meat, piece, 4 x 2 x ¼ ...... 2 pieces	85	135	25	0	3	0.9	0.5	0.7	59
Light & dark meat:									
Chopped or diced .... 1 cup	140	240	41	0	7	2.3	1.4	2.0	106
Poultry food products:									
Chicken:									
Canned, boneless .... 5 oz	142	235	31	0	11	3.1	4.5	2.5	88
Frankfurter, 10/lb .... 1 frank	45	115	6	3	9	2.5	3.8	1.8	45
Roll, light, 1 oz/slice .... 2 slices	57	90	11	1	4	1.1	1.7	0.9	28
Turkey:									
Gravy & turkey, frozen .... 5 oz	142	95	8	7	4	1.2	1.4	0.7	26
Ham, cured turkey thigh meat, 1 oz/slice .... 2 slices	57	75	11	tr	3	1.0	0.7	0.9	32
Loaf, breast meat, 8 slices/6 oz. pack .... 2 slices	42	45	10	0	1	0.2	0.2	0.1	17
Patties, breaded, battered, fried, 2.25 oz .... 1 patty	64	180	9	10	12	3.0	4.8	3.0	40
Roast, boneless, frozen, seasoned, light & dark meat, cooked ...... 3 oz	85	130	18	3	5	1.6	1.0	1.4	45

Soups, Sauces, and Gravies

Soups:

Canned, condensed:

Prepared with equal volume of milk:

Clam chowder,

Food (approximate measure)									
New England .... 1 cup	248	165	9	17	7	3.0	2.3	1.1	22
Cream of chicken .... 1 cup	248	190	7	15	11	4.6	4.5	1.6	27
Cream of mushroom .... 1 cup	248	205	6	15	14	5.1	3.0	4.6	20

Soups, Sauces, and Gravies continued

Foods	Approximate Measure	Weight	Calories	Protein	Carbohydrate	Total Fat	Fats Saturated	Mono-unsaturated	Poly-unsaturated	Cholesterol
	Portion	Grams	Calories	Grams	Grams	Grams	Grams	Grams	Grams	Milligrams
Tomato	1 cup	248	160	6	22	6	2.9	1.6	1.1	17
Prepared with equal volume of water:										
Bean with Bacon	1 cup	253	170	8	23	6	1.5	2.2	1.8	3
Beef broth, bouillon, consomme	1 cup	240	15	3	tr	1	0.3	0.2	tr	tr
Beef noodle	1 cup	244	85	5	9	3	1.1	1.2	0.5	5
Chicken noodle	1 cup	241	75	4	9	2	0.7	1.1	0.6	7
Chicken rice	1 cup	241	60	4	7	2	0.5	0.9	0.4	7
Clam chowder, Manhattan	1 cup	244	80	4	12	2	0.4	0.4	1.3	2
Cream of chicken	1 cup	244	115	3	9	7	2.1	3.3	1.5	10
Cream of mushroom	1 cup	244	130	2	9	9	2.4	1.7	4.2	2
Minestrone	1 cup	241	80	4	11	3	0.6	0.7	1.1	2
Pea, green	1 cup	250	165	9	27	3	1.4	1.0	0.4	0
Tomato	1 cup	244	85	2	17	2	0.4	0.4	1.0	0
Vegetable beef	1 cup	244	80	6	10	2	0.9	0.8	0.1	5
Vegetarian	1 cup	241	70	2	12	2	0.3	0.8	0.7	0
Dehydrated:										
Unprepared:										
Bouillon	1 pkt	6	15	1	1	1	0.3	0.2	tr	1
Onion	1 pkt	7	20	1	4	tr	0.1	0.2	tr	tr
Prepared with 6 oz water:										
Chicken noodle	1 pkt	188	40	2	6	1	0.2	0.4	0.3	6
Onion	1 pkt	184	20	1	4	tr	0.1	0.2	0.1	4
Tomato vegetable	1 pkt	189	40	1	8	1	0.3	0.2	0.1	8

Sauces:

Food	Measure								
From dry mix:									
Cheese, prepared with milk	1 cup	279	305	16	17	9.3	5.3	1.6	23
Hollandaise, prepared with water	1 cup	259	240	5	20	11.6	5.9	0.9	14
White sauce, prepared with milk	1 cup	264	240	10	13	6.4	4.7	1.7	21
From home recipe:									
White sauce, medium	1 cup	250	395	10	30	9.1	11.9	7.2	24
Ready to serve:									
Barbecue	1 Tbs	16	10	tr	tr	tr	0.1	0.1	2
Soy	1 Tbs	18	10	2	0	0.0	0.0	0.0	2

Gravies:

Food	Measure								
Canned:									
Beef	1 cup	233	125	9	5	2.7	2.3	0.2	11
Chicken	1 cup	238	190	5	14	3.4	6.1	3.6	13
Mushroom	1 cup	238	120	3	6	1.0	2.8	2.4	13
From dry mix:									
Brown	1 cup	261	80	3	2	0.9	0.8	0.1	14
Chicken	1 cup	260	85	3	2	0.5	0.9	0.4	14

Sugars and Sweets

Candy:

Food	Measure								
Caramels, plain or chocolate	1 oz	28	115	1	3	2.2	0.3	0.1	22
Chocolate:									
Milk, plain	1 oz	28	145	2	9	5.4	3.0	0.3	16
Milk, with almonds	1 oz	28	150	3	10	4.8	4.1	0.7	15
Milk, with peanuts	1 oz	28	155	4	11	4.2	3.5	1.5	13
Milk, with rice cereal	1 oz	28	140	2	7	4.4	2.5	0.2	18

Foods	Approximate Measure (Portion)	Weight (Grams)	Calories	Protein (Grams)	Carbohydrate (Grams)	Total Fat (Grams)	Fats Saturated (Grams)	Fats Mono-unsaturated (Grams)	Fats Poly-unsaturated (Grams)	Cholesterol (Milligrams)
Sugars and Sweets										
Semisweet, small pieces, 60/oz ....1 cup	170	860	7	97	61	36.2	19.9	1.9	96
Sweet (dark)................1 oz	28	150	1	16	10	5.9	3.3	0.3	16
Fondant, uncoated (mints, candy corn, other) ....1 oz	28	105	tr	27	0	0.0	0.0	0.0	27
Fudge, chocolate, plain........1 oz	28	115	1	21	3	2.1	1.0	0.1	21
Gum drops...............1 oz	28	100	tr	25	tr	tr	tr	0.1	25
Hard ....1 oz	28	110	0	28	0	0.0	0.0	0.0	0
Jelly beans ....1 oz	28	105	tr	26	tr	tr	tr	0.1	0
Marshmallows............1 oz	28	90	1	23	0	0.0	0.0	0.0	0
Custard, baked ....1 cup	265	305	14	29	15	6.8	5.4	0.7	278
Gelatin dessert prepared with gelatin powder & water ....½ cup	120	70	2	17	0	0.0	0.0	0.0	0
Honey ....1 cup	339	1,030	1	279	0	0.0	0.0	0.0	0
1 Tbs	21	65	tr	17	0	0.0	0.0	0.0	0
Jams & preserves ....1 Tbs	20	55	tr	14	tr	0.0	tr	tr	0
1 pkt	14	40	tr	10	tr	0.0	tr	tr	0
Jellies.................1 Tbs	18	50	tr	13	tr	tr	tr	tr	0
1 pkt	14	40	tr	10	tr	tr	tr	tr	0
Popsicle, 3-fl-oz.........1 pop	95	70	0	18	0	0.0	0.0	0.0	0
Puddings: Canned:										
Chocolate..............5 oz	142	205	3	30	11	9.5	0.5	0.1	1
Tapioca...............5 oz	142	160	3	28	5	4.8	tr	tr	tr
Vanilla................5 oz	142	220	2	33	10	9.5	0.2	0.1	1

Dry mix, prepared with whole milk:

Chocolate:

Food	Measure									
Instant	½ cup	130	155	4	27	4	2.3	1.1	0.2	14
Regular, cooked	½ cup	130	150	4	25	4	2.4	1.1	0.1	15
Rice	½ cup	132	155	4	27	4	2.3	1.1	0.1	15
Tapioca	½ cup	130	145	4	25	4	2.3	1.1	0.1	15

Vanilla:

Food	Measure									
Instant	½ cup	130	150	4	27	4	2.2	1.1	0.2	15
Regular	½ cup	130	145	4	25	4	2.3	1.0	0.1	15

Sugars:

Food	Measure									
Brown, pressed down	1 cup	220	820	0	212	0	0.0	0.0	0.0	0

White:

Food	Measure									
Granulated	1 cup	200	770	0	199	0	0.0	0.0	0.0	0
	1 Tbs	12	45	0	12	0	0.0	0.0	0.0	0
	1 pkt	6	25	0	6	0	0.0	0.0	0.0	0
Powdered, sifted, spooned into cup	1 cup	100	385	0	100	0	0.0	0.0	0.0	0

Syrups:

Chocolate-flavored syrup or topping:

Food	Measure									
Thin type	2 Tbs	38	85	1	22	tr	0.2	0.1	0.1	0
Fudge type	2 Tbs	38	125	2	21	5	3.1	1.7	0.2	0
Molasses, cane, blackstrap	2 Tbs	40	85	0	22	0	0.0	0.0	0.0	0
Table syrup, corn & maple	2 Tbs	42	122	0	32	0	0.0	0.0	0.0	0

Vegetable and Vegetable Products

Food	Measure									
Alfalfa seed, sprouted	1 cup	33	10	1	1	tr	tr	tr	0.1	0
Artichokes, cooked	1 art	120	55	3	12	tr	tr	tr	0.1	0

Vegetable and Vegetables Products continued

Foods	Approximate Measure (Portion)	Weight Grams	Calories Calories	Protein Grams	Carbohydrate Grams	Total Fat Grams	Fats Saturated Grams	Mono-unsaturated Grams	Poly-unsaturated Grams	Cholesterol Milligrams
Asparagus, green:										
Cooked, drained:										
From raw:										
Cuts & tips............1 cup		180	45	5	8	1	0.1	tr	0.2	0
Spears, ½" diam. at base.....4 spears		60	15	2	3	tr	tr	tr	0.1	0
From frozen:										
Cuts & tips............1 cup		180	50	5	9	1	0.2	tr	0.3	0
Spears, ½" diam. at base.....4 spears		60	15	2	3	tr	0.1	tr	0.1	0
Canned, spears, ½" diam. at base.....4 spears		80	10	1	2	tr	tr	tr	0.1	0
Bamboo shoots, canned, drained......1 cup		131	25	2	4	1	0.1	tr	0.2	0
Beans:										
Lima, immature seeds, frozen, cooked, drained:										
Thick-seeded types............1 cup		170	170	10	32	1	0.1	tr	0.3	0
Thin-seeded types ....1 cup		180	190	12	35	1	0.1	tr	0.3	0
Snap:										
Cooked, drained:										
From raw, cut & French style............1 cup		125	45	2	10	tr	0.1	tr	0.2	0
Frozen, cut............1 cup		135	35	2	8	tr	tr	tr	0.1	0
Canned, drained............cup		135	25	2	6	tr	tr	tr	0.1	0
Bean sprouts, mung:										
Raw............1 cup		104	30	3	6	tr	tr	tr	0.1	0
Cooked, drained............1 cup		124	25	3	5	tr	tr	tr	tr	0

Beets:										
Cooked, drained:										
Diced or sliced	1 cup	170	55	2	11	tr	tr	tr	tr	0
Whole, 2" diam.	2 beets	100	30	1	7	tr	tr	tr	tr	0
Canned, drained, diced or sliced	1 cup	170	55	2	12	tr	tr	tr	0.1	0
Beet greens, leaves & stems, cooked, drained	1 cup	144	40	4	8	tr	tr	0.1	0.1	0
Black-eyed peas, immature seed, cooked:										
From raw	1 cup	165	180	13	30	1	0.3	0.1	0.6	0
From frozen	1 cup	170	225	14	40	1	0.3	0.1	0.5	0
Broccoli:										
Raw	1 spear	151	40	4	8	1	0.1	tr	0.3	0
Cooked:										
From raw:										
Spear, medium	1 spear	180	50	5	10	1	0.1	tr	0.2	0
Cut in ½" pieces	1 cup	155	45	5	9	tr	0.1	tr	0.2	0
From frozen:										
Piece, 4–5" long	1 piece	30	10	1	2	tr	tr	tr	tr	0
Chopped	1 cup	185	50	6	10	tr	tr	tr	0.1	0
Brussels sprouts, cooked, drained:										
From raw, 7–8 sprouts	1 cup	155	60	4	13	1	0.2	0.1	0.4	0
From frozen	1 cup	155	65	6	13	1	0.1	tr	0.3	0
Cabbage:										
Raw, coarsely shredded or sliced	1 cup	70	15	1	4	tr	tr	tr	0.1	0
Cooked, drained	1 cup	150	30	1	7	tr	tr	tr	0.2	0
Cabbage, Chinese:										
Pak-choi, cooked	1 cup	170	20	3	3	tr	tr	tr	0.1	0
Pe-tsai, raw, 1"	1 cup	76	10	1	2	tr	tr	tr	0.1	0

Vegetable and Vegetable Products continued

Foods	Approximate Measure	Weight	Calories	Protein	Carbohydrate	Total Fat	Saturated	Mono-unsaturated	Poly-unsaturated	Cholesterol
	Portion	Grams	Calories	Grams	Grams	Grams	Grams	Grams	Grams	Milligrams
Cabbage, red, raw, coarsely shredded or sliced.....1 cup		70	20	1	4	tr	tr	tr	0.1	0
Cabbage, savoy, raw, coarsely shredded.....1 cup		70	20	1	4	tr	tr	tr	tr	0
Carrots:										
Raw, scraped:										
Whole, 7½ x 1⅛.....1 carrot		72	30	1	7	tr	tr	tr	0.1	0
Grated.....1 cup		110	45	1	11	tr	tr	tr	0.1	0
Cooked, sliced:										
From raw.....1 cup		156	70	2	16	tr	0.1	tr	0.1	0
From frozen.....1 cup		146	55	2	12	tr	tr	tr	0.1	0
Canned, sliced.....1 cup		146	35	1	8	tr	0.1	tr	0.1	0
Cauliflower:										
Raw (flowerets).....1 cup		100	25	2	5	tr	tr	tr	0.1	0
Cooked, drained:										
From raw, flowerets.....1 cup		125	30	2	6	tr	tr	tr	0.1	0
Frozen, flowerets.....1 cup		180	35	3	7	tr	0.1	tr	0.2	0
Celery, pascal type, raw:										
Stalk, large outer, 8 x 1½" at root end.....1 stalk		40	5	tr	1	tr	tr	tr	tr	0
Diced.....1 cup		120	20	1	4	tr	tr	tr	0.1	0
Collards, cooked, drained:										
From raw, leaves without stems.....1 cup		190	25	2	5	tr	0.1	tr	0.2	0
From frozen.....1 cup		170	60	5	12	1	0.1	0.1	0.4	0

Food	Measure									
Corn, sweet:										
Cooked, drained:										
From raw, ear 5 x 2"	1 ear	77	85	3	19	1	0.2	0.3	0.5	0
From frozen:										
Ear 3½" long	1 ear	63	60	2	14	tr	0.1	0.1	0.2	0
Kernels	1 cup	165	135	5	34	tr	tr	tr	0.1	0
Canned:										
Cream style	1 cup	256	185	4	46	1	0.2	0.3	0.5	0
Whole kernel	1 cup	210	165	5	41	1	0.2	0.3	0.5	0
Cucumber, with peel, slices, ⅛" thick	6 lg or 8 sm slices	28	5	tr	1	tr	tr	tr	tr	0
Dandelion greens, cooked, drained	1 cup	105	35	2	7	1	0.1	tr	0.3	0
Eggplant, cooked,	1 cup	96	25	1	6	tr	tr	tr	0.1	0
Endive, curly, raw, small pieces	1 cup	50	10	1	2	tr	tr	tr	tr	0
Jerusalem-artichoke, raw, sliced	1 cup	150	115	3	26	tr	0.0	tr	tr	0
Kale, cooked, drained:										
From raw, chopped	1 cup	130	40	2	7	1	0.1	tr	0.3	0
From frozen	1 cup	130	40	4	7	1	0.1	tr	0.3	0
Kohlrabi, thickened bulb-like stems, cooked, diced	1 cup	165	50	3	11	tr	tr	tr	0.1	0
Lettuce, raw:										
Butterhead, as Boston:										
Head, 5" diam.	1 head	163	20	2	4	tr	tr	tr	0.2	0
Leaves	1 outer or 2 inner	15	tr	tr	tr	tr	tr	tr	tr	0
Crisphead, as iceberg:										
Head, 6" diam.	1 head	539	70	5	11	1	0.1	tr	0.5	0
Wedge, ¼ of head	1 wedge	135	20	1	3	tr	tr	tr	0.1	0
Pieces, chopped	1 cup	55	5	1	1	tr	tr	tr	0.1	0

Vegetable and Vegetable Products continued

Foods	Approximate Measure / Portion	Weight / Grams	Calories / Calories	Protein / Grams	Carbohydrate / Grams	Total Fat / Grams	Fats — Saturated / Grams	Fats — Mono-unsaturated / Grams	Fats — Poly-unsaturated / Grams	Cholesterol / Milligrams
Looseleaf, bunching varieties such as romaine, chopped or shredded	1 cup	56	10	1	2	tr	tr	tr	0.1	0
Mushrooms:										
Raw, sliced	1 cup	70	20	1	3	tr	tr	tr	0.1	0
Cooked, drained	1 cup	156	40	3	8	1	0.1	tr	0.3	0
Canned, drained	1 cup	156	35	3	8	tr	0.1	tr	0.2	0
Mustard greens, without stems & midribs, cooked	1 cup	140	20	3	3	tr	tr	0.2	0.1	0
Okra pods, cooked	8 pods	85	25	2	6	tr	tr	tr	tr	0
Onions:										
Raw:										
Chopped	1 cup	160	55	2	12	tr	0.1	0.1	0.2	0
Sliced	1 cup	115	40	1	8	tr	0.1	tr	0.1	0
Cooked, whole or sliced, drained	1 cup	210	60	2	13	tr	0.1	tr	0.1	0
Onions, spring, raw, bulb, 3/8" diam. & white portion of top	6 onions	30	10	1	2	tr	tr	tr	tr	0
Onion rings, breaded, par-fried, frozen	2 rings	20	80	1	8	5	1.7	2.2	1.0	0
Parsley:										
Raw	10 sprigs	10	5	tr	1	tr	tr	tr	tr	0
Freeze-dried	1 Tbs	0.4	tr	tr	tr	tr	tr	tr	tr	0
Parsnips, cooked	1 cup	156	125	2	30	tr	0.1	0.2	0.1	0
Peas, edible pod, cooked	1 cup	160	65	5	11	tr	0.1	tr	0.2	0

Food	Measure	Grams								
Peas, green:										
Canned, drained	1 cup	170	115	8	21	1	0.1	0.1	0.3	0
Frozen, cooked	1 cup	160	125	8	23	tr	0.1	tr	0.2	0
Peppers:										
Hot chili, raw	1 pepper	45	20	1	4	tr	tr	tr	tr	0
Sweet (5/lb):										
Raw	1 pepper	74	20	1	4	tr	tr	tr	0.2	0
Cooked	1 pepper	73	15	tr	3	tr	tr	tr	0.1	0
Potatoes, cooked:										
Baked (2/lb):										
With skin	1 potato	202	220	5	51	tr	0.1	tr	0.1	0
Flesh only	1 potato	156	145	3	34	tr	tr	tr	0.1	0
Boiled (3/lb):										
Peeled after	1 potato	136	120	3	27	tr	tr	tr	0.1	0
Peeled before	1 potato	135	115	2	27	tr	tr	tr	0.1	0
French fried, frozen:										
Oven heated	10 strips	50	110	2	17	4	2.1	1.8	0.3	0
Fried in veg. oil	10 strips	50	160	2	20	8	2.5	1.6	3.8	0
Potato products, prepared:										
Au gratin:										
From dry mix	1 cup	245	230	6	31	10	6.3	2.9	0.3	12
From home mix	1 cup	245	325	12	28	19	11.6	5.3	0.7	56
Hashed brown, from frozen	1 cup	156	340	5	44	18	7.0	8.0	2.1	0
Mashed:										
From home recipe:										
Milk added	1 cup	210	160	4	37	1	0.7	0.3	0.1	4
Milk & margarine	1 cup	210	225	4	35	9	2.2	3.7	2.5	4
From dehydrated flakes (without milk), water, milk, butter & salt added	1 cup	210	235	4	32	12	7.2	3.3	0.5	29

Vegetable and Vegetable Products continued

Foods	Approximate Measure Portion	Weight Grams	Calories Calories	Protein Grams	Carbohydrate Grams	Total Fat Grams	Fats Saturated Grams	Fats Mono-unsaturated Grams	Fats Poly-unsaturated Grams	Cholesterol Milligrams
Potato salad, made with mayonnaise ....1 cup	250	360	7	28	21	3.6	6.2	9.3	170
Scalloped:									
From dry mix.................1 cup	245	230	5	31	11	6.5	3.0	0.5	27
From home recipe ....1 cup	245	210	7	26	9	5.5	2.5	0.4	29
Potato chips.................10 chips	20	105	1	10	7	1.8	1.2	3.6	0
Pumpkin:									
Cooked from raw ....1 cup	245	50	2	12	tr	0.1	tr	tr	0
Canned ....1 cup	245	85	3	20	1	0.4	0.1	tr	0
Radishes, raw ....4 radishes	18	5	tr	1	tr	tr	tr	tr	0
Sauerkraut, canned, solid and liquid ....1 cup	236	45	2	10	tr	0.1	tr	0.1	0
Seaweed:									
Kelp, raw ....1 oz	28	10	tr	3	tr	0.1	tr	tr	0
Spirulina.....................1 oz	28	80	16	7	2	0.8	0.2	0.6	0
Spinach:									
Raw, chopped ....1 cup	55	10	2	2	tr	tr	tr	0.1	0
Cooked, drained:									
From raw ....1 cup	180	40	5	7	tr	0.1	tr	0.2	0
From frozen...................1 cup	190	55	6	10	tr	0.1	tr	0.2	0
Canned, drained..............1 cup	214	50	6	7	1	0.2	tr	0.4	0
Spinach souffle ....1 cup	136	220	11	3	18	7.1	6.8	3.1	184
Squash, cooked:									
Summer, sliced ....1 cup	180	35	2	3	1	0.1	tr	0.2	0
Winter, baked, cubed ....1 cup	205	80	2	18	1	0.3	0.1	0.5	0

Food	Measure									
Sweet potatoes:										
Cooked (raw, 5 x 2"):										
Baked, then peeled	1 potato	114	115	2	28	tr	tr	tr	0.1	0
Boiled, peeled	1 potato	151	160	2	37	tr	0.1	tr	0.2	0
Candied, 2½ x 2"	1 piece	105	145	1	29	3	1.4	0.7	0.2	8
Canned:										
Solid pack, mashed	1 cup	255	260	5	59	1	0.1	tr	0.2	0
Pieces, 2¾ x 1"	1 piece	40	35	1	8	tr	tr	tr	tr	0
Tomatoes:										
Raw, 2⅗" diam	1 tomato	123	25	1	5	tr	tr	tr	0.1	0
Canned, solids & lq	1 cup	240	50	2	10	1	0.1	0.1	0.2	0
Tomato juice, canned	1 cup	244	40	2	10	tr	tr	tr	0.1	0
Tomato products, canned:										
Paste	1 cup	262	220	10	49	2	0.3	0.4	0.9	0
Puree	1 cup	250	105	4	25	tr	tr	tr	0.1	0
Sauce	1 cup	245	75	3	18	tr	0.1	0.1	0.2	0
Turnips, cooked	1 cup	156	30	1	8	tr	tr	tr	0.1	0
Turnip greens, cooked, drained:										
From raw	1 cup	144	30	2	6	tr	0.1	tr	0.1	0
From frozen, chopped	1 cup	164	50	5	8	1	0.2	tr	0.3	0
Vegetable juice cocktail, canned	1 cup	242	45	2	11	tr	tr	tr	0.1	0
Vegetables, mixed:										
Canned, drained	1 cup	163	75	4	15	tr	0.1	tr	0.2	0
Frozen, cooked	1 cup	182	105	5	24	tr	0.1	tr	0.1	0
Waterchestnuts	1 cup	140	70	1	17	tr	tr	tr	tr	0

Miscellaneous

Foods	Approximate Measure Portion	Weight Grams	Calories Calories	Protein Grams	Carbohydrate Grams	Total Fat Grams	Fats Saturated Grams	Mono-unsaturated Grams	Poly-unsaturated Grams	Cholesterol Milligrams
Baking powders for home use:										
Sodium aluminum sulfate:										
With monocalcium phosphate monohydrate ... 1 tsp	3	5	tr	1	0	0.0	0.0	0.0	0	
With monocalcium phosphate monohydrate, calcium sulfate ... 1 tsp	2.9	5	tr	1	0	0.0	0.0	0.0	0	
Straight phosphate ... 1 tsp	3.8	5	tr	1	0	0.0	0.0	0.0	0	
Low sodium ... 1 tsp	4.3	5	tr	1	0	0.0	0.0	0.0	0	
Catsup ... 1 cup	273	290	5	69	1	0.2	0.2	0.4	0	
1 Tbs	15	15	tr	4	tr	tr	tr	tr	0	
Celery seed ... 1 tsp	2	10	tr	1	1	tr	0.3	0.1	0	
Chili powder ... 1 tsp	2.6	10	tr	1	tr	0.1	0.1	0.2	0	
Chocolate:										
Bitter or baking ... 1 oz	28	145	3	8	15	9.0	4.9	0.5	0	
Semisweet, see Candy										
Cinnamon ... 1 tsp	2.3	5	tr	2	tr	tr	tr	tr	0	
Curry powder ... 1 tsp	2	5	tr	1	tr	—	—	—	0	
Garlic powder ... 1 tsp	2.8	10	tr	2	tr	tr	tr	tr	0	
Gelatin, dry ... 1 pkt	7	25	6	0	tr	tr	tr	tr	0	
Mustard, prepared ... 1 tsp	5	5	tr	tr	tr	tr	0.2	tr	0	
Olives, canned:										
Green ... 4 med or 3 x-lg	13	15	tr	tr	2	0.2	1.2	0.1	0	
Ripe, Mission ... 3 sm or 2 lg	9	15	tr	tr	2	0.3	1.3	0.2	0	

Food	Measure	(g)								
Onion powder	1 tsp	2.1	5	tr	2	tr	tr	tr	tr	0
Oregano	1 tsp	1.5	5	tr	1	tr	tr	tr	0.1	0
Paprika	1 tsp	2.1	5	tr	1	tr	tr	tr	0.2	0
Pepper black	1 tsp	2.1	5	tr	1	tr	tr	tr	tr	0
Pickles, cucumber:										
Dill, 3¾ x 1¼″	1 pickle	65	5	tr	1	tr	tr	tr	0.1	0
Fresh pack, slices 1½ x ¼″	2 slices	15	10	tr	3	tr	tr	tr	tr	0
Sweet gherkin, small	1 pickle	15	20	tr	5	tr	tr	tr	tr	0
Relish, finely chopped, sweet	1 Tbs	15	20	tr	5	0	tr	tr	tr	0
Salt	1 tsp	5.5	0	0	0	0	0.0	0.0	0.0	0
Vinegar, cider	1 Tbs	15	tr	tr	1	0	0.0	0.0	0.0	0
Yeast:										
Baker's, dry active	1 pkg	7	20	3	3	tr	tr	0.1	tr	0
Brewer's dry	1 Tbs	8	25	3	3	tr	tr	tr	0.0	0

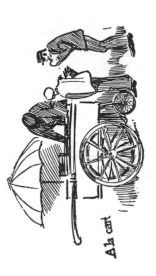

A la cart

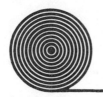

ORDER YOUR COPY(S) TODAY!

___ THE LOW BLOOD SUGAR HANDBOOK (Revised edition) $12.95
copy(s)

___ THE LOW BLOOD SUGAR COOKBOOK $12.95
copy(s)

___ THE LOW BLOOD SUGAR CASSETTE (1 hour) .... $ 9.95
copy(s)

___ VITAL HEALTH FACTS and COMPOSITION OF FOODS .... $ 4.50
copy(s)

___ CHOLESTEROL LOWERING AND CONTROLLING
copy(s) 3 WEEK PLAN: HANDBOOK & COOKBOOK $12.95

Send check or money order to: **Franklin Publishers, Box 1338, Bryn Mawr, PA 19010.**
For total order, include $2.00 for postage and handling or $3.00 for 1st class postage
and handling.   PA residents, include state sales tax.

Orders outside of U.S. must be paid in U.S. dollars with a Postal Money Order.

Send to:

Mr./Ms. _____
(Print or type)

Address_____

City_____ State_____ Zip_____

Phone number _____
Price subject to change without notice.

ORDER YOUR COPY(S) TODAY!

___ THE LOW BLOOD SUGAR HANDBOOK (Revised edition) $12.95
copy(s)

___ THE LOW BLOOD SUGAR COOKBOOK $12.95
copy(s)

___ THE LOW BLOOD SUGAR CASSETTE (1 hour) .... $ 9.95
copy(s)

___ VITAL HEALTH FACTS and COMPOSITION OF FOODS ...... $ 4.50
copy(s)

___ CHOLESTEROL LOWERING AND CONTROLLING
copy(s) 3 WEEK PLAN: HANDBOOK & COOKBOOK $12.95

Send check or money order to: **Franklin Publishers, Box 1338, Bryn Mawr, PA 19010.**
For total order, include $2.00 for postage and handling or $3.00 for 1st class postage
and handling.   PA residents, include state sales tax.

Orders outside of U.S. must be paid in U.S. dollars with a Postal Money Order.

Send to:

Mr./Ms. _____
(Print or type)

Address_____

City_____ State_____ Zip_____

Phone number _____
Price subject to change without notice.

ORDER YOUR COPY(S) TODAY!

____ THE LOW BLOOD SUGAR HANDBOOK (Revised edition) $12.95
copy(s)

____ THE LOW BLOOD SUGAR COOKBOOK $12.95
copy(s)

____ THE LOW BLOOD SUGAR CASSETTE (1 hour) .... $ 9.95
copy(s)

____ VITAL HEALTH FACTS and COMPOSITION OF FOODS....... $ 4.50
copy(s)

____ CHOLESTEROL LOWERING AND CONTROLLING
copy(s) 3 WEEK PLAN: HANDBOOK & COOKBOOK $12.95

Send check or money order to: **Franklin Publishers, Box 1338, Bryn Mawr, PA 19010.**
For total order, include $2.00 for postage and handling or $3.00 for 1st class postage
and handling.   PA residents, include state sales tax.

Orders outside of U.S. must be paid in U.S. dollars with a Postal Money Order.

Send to:

Mr./Ms. _____
         (Print or type)

Address_____

City_____ State_____ Zip_____

Phone number _____
                    Price subject to change without notice.

ORDER YOUR COPY(S) TODAY!

____ THE LOW BLOOD SUGAR HANDBOOK (Revised edition) $12.95
copy(s)

____ THE LOW BLOOD SUGAR COOKBOOK $12.95
copy(s)

____ THE LOW BLOOD SUGAR CASSETTE (1 hour) .... $ 9.95
copy(s)

____ VITAL HEALTH FACTS and COMPOSITION OF FOODS....... $ 4.50
copy(s)

____ CHOLESTEROL LOWERING AND CONTROLLING
copy(s) 3 WEEK PLAN: HANDBOOK & COOKBOOK $12.95

Send check or money order to: **Franklin Publishers, Box 1338, Bryn Mawr, PA 19010.**
For total order, include $2.00 for postage and handling or $3.00 for 1st class postage
and handling.   PA residents, include state sales tax.

Orders outside of U.S. must be paid in U.S. dollars with a Postal Money Order.

Send to:

Mr./Ms. _____
         (Print or type)

Address_____

City_____ State_____ Zip_____

Phone number _____
                    Price subject to change without notice.

To order, send note or copy of order form with payment

ORDER YOUR COPY(S) TODAY!

Please send:

_____ **THE LOW BLOOD SUGAR HANDBOOK (Revised Edition)**
copy(s) *By Edward & Patricia Krimmel* $12.95
Highly praised by Harvey Ross, M.D., this is a new upscaled approach to the diagnosis and treatment of hypoglycemia (low blood sugar), written with the insight and practicality that only a sufferer could have, but backed up by meticulous research and medical accuracy. The book of solutions! 192 pages

_____ **THE LOW BLOOD SUGAR COOKBOOK**
copy(s) *By Patricia & Edward Krimmel* $12.95
A very special collection of over 200 sugarless natural food recipes. Snacks to gourmet dishes designed specifically for the hypoglycemic, but which everyone can enjoy and are also valuable to diabetics and weight watchers. No artificial sweeteners or white flour are used in the recipes. Only fruit and fruit juices are used as sweeteners. 192 pages

_____ **THE LOW BLOOD SUGAR CASSETTE**
copy(s) *By Edward & Patricia Krimmel* $9.95
A one (1) hour interview conceptualizing many of the most important questions and answers pertaining to low blood sugar. Receive the feeling of personal contact with the authors.

_____ **VITAL HEALTH FACTS and COMPOSITION OF FOODS**... $4.50
copy(s) *By Edward & Patricia Krimmel*
Aids you in knowing calorie and saturated fat content of foods, your vitamin, mineral and calorie requirements and how to exercise. With this information you can control your weight, fat intake and cholesterol level all of which lead to better health. Over 100 toll free phone numbers for health information and support.

_____ **CHOLESTEROL LOWERING AND CONTROLLING 3 WEEK**
copy(s) **PLAN: HANDBOOK & COOKBOOK**
By Patricia & Edward Krimmel $12.95
Tells how to be properly tested, finger stick is not test of choice. Do you know which foods to avoid and why, and which foods to eat and why? What about weight reduction? Do you want to understand how to lose weight correctly and easily for a lifetime? Do you know which oils should be used and which ones to avoid and how to decrease the amount of saturated fat you eat? All these issues and many, many more are covered in clear, easy to understand language for a lifetime of benefit. A physician recommended book of vital information and tasty recipes.

Send check or money order to **Franklin Publishers, Box 1338, Bryn Mawr, PA 19010**. For total order, include $2.00 for postage and handling or $3.00 for 1st class postage and handling.   PA residents, include state sales tax.
Orders outside of U.S. must be paid in U.S. dollars with a Postal Money Order.

Send to:

Mr./Ms. _____
(Print or type)

Address_____

City_____ State_____ Zip_____

Phone number _____
Price subject to change without notice.

ABOUT THE AUTHORS

Patricia and Edward Krimmel are medical researchers and writers who have a special aptitude and spirit for relating very well to those trying to solve health problems. Because of their backgrounds, they are especially well equipped to write and design books dealing with solutions rather than simply talking about the problems.

Pat and Ed are known nationally within personal health care circles as true "authorities". They are the authors of the best-sellers; The Low Blood Sugar Handbook, The Low Blood Sugar Cookbook and The Cholesterol Lowering and Controlling Handbook & Cookbook. They are frequent guests on radio and television shows from coast to coast and lecture at colleges and health seminars.

Pat has her BSN from the University of Pennsylvania, has worked in childbirth education (CEA) and public health and has been maternal and infant care coordinator at the Medical College of Pennsylvania.

Ed has his degree in Social Science from St. Joseph's University, is director of HELP, The Institute for Body Chemistry and does nutritional counseling.

HEALTH TIP

Carry Medical ID

Make your own medical information card to carry in your wallet. Include your name, address, phone number, person to call in an emergency, your doctor's name & phone number, blood type, allergies (to drugs, insect bites, foods, etc.), medical conditions, and any required medications.

Wear a medical ID bracelet or necklace, it may be more easily noticed in an emergency than a card in your wallet.

Join Medic Alert which will supply a bracelet or necklace and a ID card. They have a toll-free, 24 hour emergency hotline that provides hospitals with your complete medical history. Call 1-800-432-5378 for more information.